Multi-Drug Resistance in Cancer

Scrivener Publishing
100 Cummings Center, Suite 541J
Beverly, MA 01915-6106

Publishers at Scrivener
Martin Scrivener (martin@scrivenerpublishing.com)
Phillip Carmical (pcarmical@scrivenerpublishing.com)

Multi-Drug Resistance in Cancer

Mechanism and Treatment Strategies

Rishabha Malviya, Arun Kumar Singh and Deepika Yadav

Department of Pharmacy, School of Medical and Allied Sciences, Galgotias University, India

Scrivener Publishing

WILEY

This edition first published 2023 by John Wiley & Sons, Inc., 111 River Street, Hoboken, NJ 07030, USA and Scrivener Publishing LLC, 100 Cummings Center, Suite 541J, Beverly, MA 01915, USA

For more information about Scrivener publications please visit www.scrivenerpublishing.com.

Wiley Global Headquarters
111 River Street, Hoboken, NJ 07030, USA

For details of our global editorial offices, customer services, and more information about Wiley products visit us at www.wiley.com.

Library of Congress Cataloging-in-Publication Data

ISBN 978-1-394-20921-7

Cover image: Pixabay.com
Cover design by Russell Richardson

Set in size of 11pt and Minion Pro by Manila Typesetting Company, Makati, Philippines

This book is dedicated to all healthcare professionals.
Our love for the profession shall live forever.

Contents

Foreword

Dr. Rishabha Malviya is known to me through his research and publications. I am glad to write the Foreword for this book. This is an excellent book on one of the topics which is directly related to the health of people in all countries. The title of the book is self-explanatory "*Multi-Drug Resistance in Cancer: Mechanism and Treatment Strategies*". One of the most common ways to treat cancer is with chemotherapy, but this approach is severely hampered by multi-drug resistance, which occurs when cancer cells develop resistance to a wide variety of drugs with different structures and mechanisms of action. This book examines the underlying biology of cancer drug resistance and offers fresh approaches for combating the problem. Many pathways by which cancer cells acquire the ability to resist multiple drugs have been identified over the past three decades. In addition, the development of agents or strategies to overcome resistance has been the subject of intense study. Overexpression of ATP binding cassette drug transporters like P-glycoprotein, multi-drug resistance proteins (MRPs), and breast cancer resistance proteins are just some of the topics covered in this book, along with drug ratio dependent antagonism and the paradigm of cancer stem cells. A variety of methods, such as the creation of compounds that block drug transporter function and the regulation of transporter expression, are outlined in the book as means of overcoming multi-drug resistance. Methods for studying drug resistance in animal models, techniques for detecting and imaging drug transporters, and approaches for gauging the effectiveness of resistance reversal agents can all be found within the covers of this book. This book is written for researchers at both the bench and in the clinic who are interested in the mechanisms and strategies for overcoming cancer's multi-drug resistance. The technical depth and information in this book will, in my belief, be helpful for healthcare professionals in preventing the emergence of multi-drug resistance in cancer therapy.

Prof. (Dr.) Kamla Pathak
Dean, Faculty of Pharmacy
Uttar Pradesh University of Medical Sciences,
Saifai, Etawah,
Uttar Pradesh, India

Preface

Cancer is a major killer all over the world. Even with all the progress made, chemotherapy is the mainstay of modern cancer treatment and still the gold standard. The progression of cellular defeat of numerous independent anticancer drugs in terms of their chemical structure is a major barrier to successful chemotherapy. Multi-drug resistance (MDR) is a term for the fact that most cancer patients exhibit this phenomenon. According to the numbers, drug resistance carries the blame for ninety percent of cancer patient deaths. Refractory cancer and tumour recurrence are common outcomes of prolonged chemotherapy Because of the prevalence of drug-resistance mutations, the difficulty of treating tumours increases and the therapeutic efficacy of drugs decreases.

This book covers a wide range of topics related to multi-drug resistance, from drug ratio-dependent antagonism and cancer stem cells to overexpression of ATP-binding cassette drug carrier like P-glycoprotein, multidrug resistant proteins and breast cancer resistant proteins. Multi-drug resistance can be overcome by developing elements which resist drug carrier activity or modulating transporter expression. This book is an effort to keep the reader abreast of the most recent findings regarding the methods of cellular defence to current agents that fight against cancer. It should help direct future research toward the discovery of more efficient approaches to cancer treatment by elucidating the methods of MDR and the intended recipients of novel chemotherapeutic agents.

MDR in Cancer: Mechanism & Treatment Strategies, has 9 chapters on topics such as, autophagy and drug resistance, efflux transporters, drug transporter expression, breast cancer resistance to targeted therapies, advances in metallodrug-driven combination cancer treatment, and using natural agents to overcome cancer tolerance to drugs. Chapter 1 outlines treatment strategies for MDR in cancer. In Chapter 2, the various methods that contribute to cancer tolerance to drugs and the novel strategies to overcome multi-drug resistance are described. The molecular systems for the treatment of drug addiction-resistant cancer cells and natural products for the clinical management of drug resistance in these cells are the primary topics of discussion in Chapters 3 and 4, respectively. Defeating multi-drug resistance (MDR) through autophagy and using transport inhibitors to better the clinical outcome of colorectal cancer are topics covered in the next two chapters. Substantial contributions of epithelial-mesenchymal transitions to resistance to cancer drug therapy are discussed in Chapter 7. The evolution of metal-based drugs is covered in detail in Chapter 8, and the book concludes with a final chapter presenting a number of novel approaches for halting the emergence of multi-drug resistance in breast cancer. This book is written for researchers at both the bench and in the clinic who are interested in the mechanisms and strategies for overcoming cancer's multi-drug resistance.

The Authors
May 2023

Acknowledgment

When I started working on book writing, the first topic that came to mind was cancer, but I was afraid because it was a challenging task. But now that I have finally worked on the subject, I find it has been a very pleasant experience. It is, by far, more rewarding and motivating than what I had imagined. At the outset, I would like to begin by expressing our gratitude to the Almighty, whose unending blessing and supreme power enable us to accomplish all of our goals.

Although this phase in my life was full of ups and downs, I will always be thankful to my family for their unwavering support and encouragement, which allowed me to accomplish this work.

I want to express my gratitude to the management of Galgotias University for motivating me for research and recognizing my potential, and for inspiring me every day.

I would like to express my deepest gratitude to Miss. Sonali Sundram, Faculty, Department of Pharmacy, Galgotias University, India for her continuous motivation and support. Her enthusiasm for hard work and dedication toward work always inspires me.

Many thanks to my students (undergraduate and postgraduate), colleagues and all the co-authors for being part of this book, because without their participation, the writing of this book would not have been completed.

Lastly, I would like to thank our publisher for their support, innovative suggestions, and guidance in bringing out this edition.

Rishabha Malviya
May 2023

1

Multi-Drug Resistance in Cancer: Understanding of Treatment Strategies

Rishabha Malviya*, **Arun Kumar Singh and Deepika Yadav**

Abstract

In the United States, cancer is the second largest killer. Surgery, cytotoxic chemotherapy, targeted therapy, radiation therapy, endocrine therapy, and immunotherapy are among the most important therapies for cancer management. Resistance to conventional chemotherapeutic agents and/or innovative targeted medications remains a significant challenge in cancer treatment despite decades of effort and progress. Cancer relapses are a leading cause of mortality, and they are often the result of either preexisting drug resistance (intrinsic) or the development of new drug resistance (acquired). Drug resistance is more difficult to manage due to the heterogeneity of people and tumors, as well as cancer's adaptability in evading therapy. To better direct future cancer therapy and boost outcomes, a better understanding of the factors that contribute to drug resistance is required. In this synopsis, examination of both innate and acquired forms of resistance. In addition, new information about the mechanisms of drug resistance will be presented and discussed. The details of recent findings that highlight the role of ATP in drug resistance, including the presence of extremely high levels of extracellular ATP within tumors and the importation of extracellular ATP into tumor cells from the environment has been discussed here. Due to the complex nature of drug resistance, it is possible that combining and customizing treatments for cancer patients may be the most effective strategy for combating the disease.

Keywords: Cancer, drug resistance, heterogeneity of tumor, combination therapy, acquired resistance

1.1 Introduction

To put it simply, cancer is the second largest killer in the United States [1]. A total of 1.7 million persons were diagnosed with cancer in 2017,

**Corresponding author:* rishabhamalviya19@gmail.com

Rishabha Malviya, Arun Kumar Singh and Deepika Yadav. Multi-Drug Resistance in Cancer: Mechanism and Treatment Strategies, (1–30) © 2023 Scrivener Publishing LLC

with 0.6 million succumbing to the disease [2]. Up to 90% of cancer-related fatalities are caused by medication resistance and the ensuing ineffectiveness of treatment [3–7]. The mechanism of drug resistance against cancerous cells is illustrated in Figure 1.1.

Cancer cells that have acquired tolerance to pharmacological therapy are said to have developed drug resistance. Many different physiological and molecular pathways, including mutations and epigenetic alterations in cancer cells, upregulation of a previously conserved drug efflux pump, and others, contribute to the development of resistance to anticancer treatments.

Surgical resection, cytotoxic chemotherapy, targeted therapy, radiotherapy, irradiation, hormone therapy, and immunotherapy are now the cornerstones of cancer management [8–12]. Although there have been great strides achieved in cancer treatment over the last several decades, relapses a leading cause of cancer deaths are still often the result of the body's resistance to chemotherapy or targeted medications. Many traditional chemotherapeutic anticancer medicines work by directly altering the DNA of cancer cells to destroy them. This method is inherently non-specific and

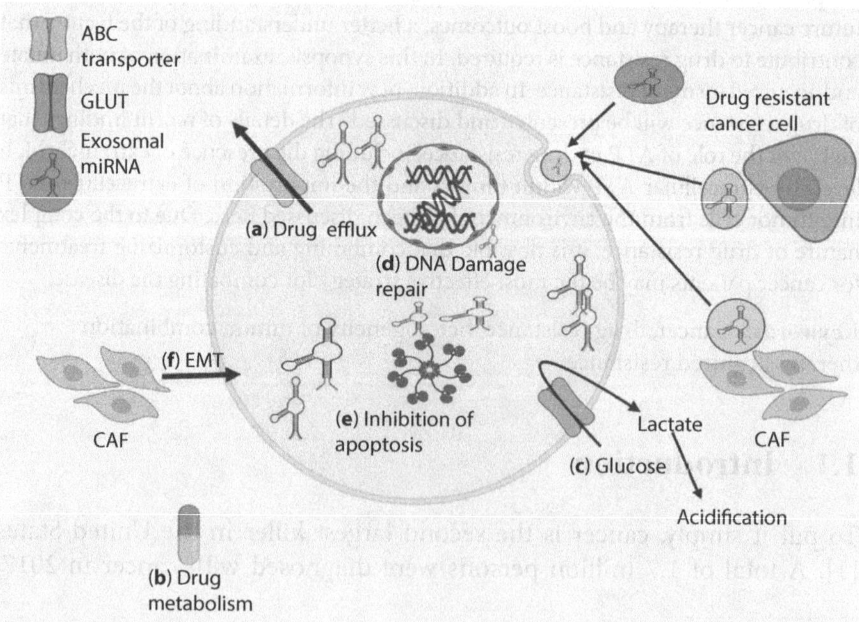

Figure 1.1 Diagrammatic representation of cancerous cells developing resistance against the drug.

may have severe side effects in certain patients. Many new medications that specifically target or inhibit cancer-promoting alterations have been produced in the last few decades. While the earliest stages of therapy with these medications may have spectacular outcomes, the vast majority of patients will eventually develop resistance. To provide just one example, between 30% and 55% of individuals with non-small cell lung cancer (NSCLC) have a recurrence and ultimately succumb to the disease [13]. Recurrence of ovarian adenocarcinoma is common, occurring in 50% to 70% of cases within a year following surgery and chemotherapy [14]. About 20 % of juvenile acute lymphoblastic leukemia patients suffer recurrence [15].

Better knowledge of the processes behind the formation of drug resistance is critically required and will help to develop innovative treatment options and lead to better clinical results. This chapter will explain what drug resistance is and how it may be acquired or developed, as well as highlight recent findings on the causes of drug resistance and address novel approaches to combating drug resistance and enhancing the effectiveness of anticancer drugs.

1.2 Both Congenital and Developed Resistance to Drugs

The development of drug resistance may be classified as either innate or acquired. About half of all cancer patients with drug resistance have intrinsic resistance, which occurs before medication treatment, and 50 % have acquired resistance, which is produced by therapy [16, 17].

1.2.1 Intrinsic Resistance

For medications to have less of an effect, they must overcome the patient's natural resistance to them, which is known as "intrinsic resistance." (1) Preexisting (inherent) genetic mutations in the majority of tumors lead to decreased responsiveness of cancer cells, such as triple-negative breast cancer cells, to both chemo and target drugs; (2) heterogeneity of tumors in which preexisting insensitive subpopulations, including cancer stem cells, will be selected upon drug treatment, resulting in a relapse in later stages of treatment; (3) activation of intrigue resistant pathways (such as anticancer drugs).

Preexisting genetic mutation(s) of genes involved in cancer cell proliferation and/or apoptosis may cause cancer cells to be intrinsically resistant to drugs. Overexpression of HER2 has been linked to a worse response to cisplatin in patients with gastric cancer [18]. Increased resistance to chemotherapy is achieved by a process called epithelial-mesenchymal transition (EMT), which is triggered by increased HER2 gene expression by upregulating the transcription factor Snail. It was also discovered that the survival rate of HER2/Snail double-positive patients was lower than that of single-positive or double-negative patients.

EMT, resistance to p53-induced apoptosis, and a self-renewal drive were all demonstrated to be mediated by the transcriptional repressors Snail and Slug [19]. These two processes provide radiation and chemotherapeutic resistance to cancer stem cells (CSCs). Resistant cells have also been demonstrated to have greater mesenchymal characteristics [20, 21]. These parallel alterations establish a connection between inherent drug resistance, EMT, and CSCs.

Relapse after chemotherapeutic therapy may also be caused by preexisting resistant subpopulations in malignancies. Increasing data indicate that intratumoral genetic variability in primary cancers exists prior to therapeutic intervention [22–24]. The majority of tumor cells are vulnerable to the medicine; therefore, patients would initially react to treatment. After pharmacological therapy, however, the resistant subclones would multiply and produce a relapse [25–27]. This inherent drug resistance is sometimes misunderstood as acquired resistance since the tumor would initially shrink during treatment, leading many to believe that the resistance was gained as a result of therapy. Cancer stem cells (CSCs) are a self-renewing and differentiating subset of tumor cells that contribute to tumor development [28]. Multiple cancer types, including leukemia [29], glioblastoma [30], and pancreatic cancer [31], have documented their involvement in chemotherapeutic treatment resistance. It is possible that medication resistance may only be mitigated by the use of a combination treatment that simultaneously eliminates CSCs and the bulk of the tumor.

Anticancer medications are no exception; activation of intrinsic mechanisms intended to defend against environmental contaminants might decrease their therapeutic effects. ATP binding cassette (ABC) transporter-mediated drug efflux [32] and the glutathione (GSH)/glutathione S-transferase system are examples of such defence systems that operate to either decrease drug accumulation in cells or detoxify drug-treated cancer cells, respectively [33].

1.2.2 Acquired Resistance

Slowly diminishing anticancer activity after pharmacological therapy is a hallmark of acquired resistance. Tumor microenvironmental (TME) alterations, mutations in therapeutic targets, and secondary oncogene activation are all potential causes of acquired resistance.

Tumors that have been reduced in size may regain growth capability if they develop resistance to treatment. Eight patients with acute myeloid leukemia had their genetic profiles examined using whole-genome sequencing before and after relapse [34]. Genome-wide analysis of primary and recurrent cancers revealed previously unknown alterations in genes. Furthermore, the data demonstrated an increase in transversion mutations in recurrent tumors, which may indicate that DNA damage in cancer cells produced by cytotoxic chemotherapeutic treatments enhanced the likelihood of the development of new mutations.

When mutations or changes in the expression levels of the genes-producing target proteins occur in cancer cells, the cells may become resistant to the therapeutic effects of the medications. As an example of a secondary mutation inside the target kinase, the threonine 315 to isoleucine (T315I) mutation in the BCR-ABL kinase domain is a case in point. Although the BCR-ABL tyrosine kinase inhibitor (TKI) imatinib is widely used to treat chronic myelogenous leukemia, between 20% and 30% of individuals develop resistance to the drug or relapse following treatment [35]. The resistance may be explained, in part, by a point mutation in the fusion tyrosine kinase protein, T315I, which prevents it from functioning properly [35–37]. By replacing threonine 315 with isoleucine, the drug's effectiveness is greatly diminished because the ATP-binding site of BCR-ABL no longer forms a hydrogen bond with imatinib.

The dynamic variations in TME during therapy may potentially lead to the development of drug resistance. Tumor cells and their microenvironment engage in cross-talk throughout disease progression and resistance. The interaction involves exosomes secreted by both cancer and stromal cells. Cancer cells and tumor-associated macrophages (TAMs) in the TME rely on exosomes, which are generated by cancer cells and contain specific miRNAs, to interact with one another, according to the research [38]. Neuroblastoma (NBL) tumor cells secrete exosomic miR-21, which stimulates tumor-associated macrophages (TAMs) to generate exosomic miR-155, which then silences the TERF1 gene in NBL cells. Increased telomerase activity and tolerance to chemotherapy would arise from reduced expression of TERF1, a protein that inhibits telomerase. As a result, drug resistance may be facilitated by the exchanging of exosomal miRNAs between tumor cells and stromal cells in the TME.

While tumors develop and are treated, the innate and acquired resistance mechanisms discussed above might coexist. There may be significant differences between the underlying mechanisms of intrinsic drug resistance and those of acquired drug resistance. Also possible is a gradual increase in the organism's innate resistance to drugs. The susceptibility of individual cancer cells to a certain treatment is determined beforehand by the extent to which those cells exhibit inherent drug resistance. It is important to rule out the possibility of medication resistance by conducting genomic and other biochemical tests before designing the treatment strategy. Adjustments to treatment plans are necessary when acquired medication resistance has emerged.

One goal of cancer medication therapy should be to halt tumor development without triggering acquired, or at least unmanageable, drug resistance. Acquired drug resistance is a serious problem that has to be addressed in any effective drug treatment approach.

1.3 Drug-Resistance Mechanisms

Although differentiating between innate and acquired resistance is vital from a scientific standpoint, the particular mechanisms of resistance are more relevant from a therapeutic perspective.

1.3.1 Increased Efflux of Drugs

It has been hypothesized that reduced intracellular drug accumulation as a result of increased anticancer agent efflux is the primary cause of chemotherapy resistance [7, 39, 40]. Excessive drug efflux rates may indicate innate or acquired resistance, depending on whether the problem appears before or after drug treatment.

The ABC transporter superfamily is the most common source of transmembrane transporters involved in drug efflux. There are 48 ABC genes in the human genome, and these genes have been divided into seven different subfamilies (ABCA-ABCG) [41, 42]. Among them, ABCB1, ABCC1, and ABCG2 play significant roles in the development of MDR to cancer chemotherapy.

Too far, ABCB1 (also known as MDR1 or P-gp) has been one of the best-studied ABC transporters. It consists of two nucleotide-binding domains that bind and hydrolyze ATP and two transmembrane domains that establish a passage for substrates. Transport substrates are pumped out as a result of conformational changes in the transporter that occur in conjunction with ATP binding and hydrolysis [43]. Etoposide, doxorubicin, paclitaxel, and vinblastine are only some of the many substrates that may be bound and pumped out of the cell by ABCB1 due to its many drug binding sites [44–48]. Numerous tumor forms, including kidney, lung, liver, colon, and rectum, have been shown to display high levels of ABCB1 prior to chemotherapy [49]. In contrast, numerous hematological malignancies, including AML and ALL, showed initially modest expression of ABCB1, followed by a substantial rise in expression of ABCB1 after chemotherapy [50–52].

ABCC1, also known as multi-drug resistance-associated protein 1 (MRP1), is responsible for the secretion of several different classes of anticancer drugs, including vinca alkaloids, anthracyclines, epipodophyllotoxins, camptothecins, and methotrexate [53]. Transported by ABCB1 include amphipathic and lipid-soluble molecules, whereas organic anionic substrates such as those conjugated to glutathione, glucuronide, or sulphate are pumped by ABCC1 [54–56]. ABCC1 overexpression has been linked to resistance in a variety of malignancies, including lung, breast, and prostate cancers [53, 57, 58].

In breast cancer, the protein ABCG2 (breast cancer resistance protein) is the primary drug efflux transporter responsible for the disease's resistance to treatment. Some malignancies have been linked to ABCG2, a gene responsible for the so-called bystander population impact. A wide variety of medicines, including chemotherapeutics (mitoxantrone, bisantrene, epipodophyllotoxin, camptothecins, flavopiridol, and anthracyclines) and TKIs (imatinib and gefitinib), are transported by this transporter [48, 59, 60]. Overexpression of ABCG2 has been identified in a wide variety of cancers, including breast cancer, lung cancer, and leukemia [60, 61].

Additional insights into the mechanisms of drug resistance have been gleaned from studies of the substrates and activities of other ABC transporters involved in tumor resistance to anticancer drugs [62]. Overexpression of ABC transporter genes, such as ABCC2 and ABCC3, causes multi-drug resistance [62–65]. These genes are responsible for transporting a wide variety of chemotherapeutic medicines, including cisplatin, doxorubicin, and etoposide. ABC transporter mutations and overexpression have a direct impact on tumor sensitivity and the therapeutic value of anticancer medicines. Better medication selection and treatment results need an accurate and comprehensive expression profile of ABC transporters in malignancies.

1.3.2 Impact on Medication Target

Targeted treatments may impede the growth of cancer cells by blocking the action of particular target proteins involved in tumor formation, making them more selective and effective to cancer cells and less destructive to normal developing cells than typical chemotherapies. However, resistance may also emerge as an issue with targeted treatment, as a consequence of changes to medication targets. Secondary mutations in the target protein or changes in expression levels as a result of epigenetic modifications are two possible causes of medication target changes.

The epidermal growth factor receptor (EGFR) TKIs erlotinib and gefitinib, which are used to treat NSCLC, have reportedly shown a high response rate at the start of treatment [66, 67]. However, within a year, over half of the responding patients would have a T790M mutation on EGFR, leading to resistance to the first and second generations of TKIs [68–70]. The alteration in EGFR conformation brought about by the threonine-to-methionine mutation increased ATP binding affinity and decreased gefitinib/erlotinib binding to the kinase [70, 71]. Third-generation TKIs, such as osimertinib and rociletinib, have been developed and shown to have therapeutic effectiveness with patients having the T790M mutation [72, 73], hence overcoming the resistance conferred by this mutation. Resistance to third-generation inhibitors develops quickly, however, therefore developing fourth-generation TKIs is essential. The C797S mutation in EGFR has been identified as a potential mechanism of the novel resistance [74]. The binding of third-generation TKIs to EGFR is hindered by the absence of the cysteine residue, which is critical for TKIs to target the ATP site. As a result, EAI045, a fourth-generation TKI that targets both T790M and C797S, was developed to bind an allosteric site on EGFR to avoid the mechanism patterns of resistance seen with the first three generations of TKIs, all of which bind to the ATP sites [75, 76]. In the never-ending fight against drug resistance, a new trend may emerge the competition between the creation of new genetic mutations and the creation of new TKIs that restore drug sensitivity.

Such a case in which resistance is produced by a change in the therapeutic target is the creation and usage of oestrogen receptor inhibitors in the treatment of breast cancer. Commonly prescribed to those with ER-positive breast cancer, tamoxifen (TAM) works by competing with oestrogen for the ligand-binding site of ER. However, medication resistance is often developed after prolonged exposure to TAM. Mutations in the ER gene and decreased ER expression levels are two examples of resistance mechanisms that may occur in individual cases [77, 78]. Aromatase inhibitors (AIs) were created as a solution to the issues with TAM and the need for new medications. These treatments act by blocking the last stage in the production of oestrogen. In postmenopausal women with hormone receptor-positive breast cancer, third-generation AIs are increasingly employed as first-line therapy [79].

1.3.3 Improved DNA-Damage Repair

Chemotherapy medications, such as cisplatin and 5-fluorouracil (5-FU), cause cancer cells to die through DNA damage. Due to DNA lesion repairs, afflicted cells' DNA damage response (DDR) to anti-cancer treatments may impair the medications' effectiveness, leading to resistance [80]. For instance, 5-FU–resistant human colon cancer cell lines were discovered to have an upregulation of DNA repair genes, such as FEN1, FANCG, and RAD23B [81, 82]. Treatment with 5-FU led to the overexpression of genes involved in DNA damage response and repair that are p53 target genes. Cell cycle arrest and apoptosis were at lower levels in resistant cell lines compared to parental cell lines due to the successful healing of the damage [82].

While DNA damage response (DDR) downregulation might alleviate resistance caused by DNA repair, it also raises the prospect of acquiring additional mutations owing to genomic instability, the accumulation of which can spark a new cycle of carcinogenesis. As a result, the DNA damage response is a mechanism involved in cancer therapy and recurrence that needs careful examination before being employed as a therapeutic target in the fight against cancer.

1.4 Senescence Escape

Cellular senescence is defined as the permanent halt in cell growth that often results in the activation of tumor suppressive mechanisms controlled by p53 and/or p16INK4a [83]. Excessive mitogenic signaling from activated oncogenes, telomere shortening [84], and non-telomeric DNA damage from chemotherapeutic medicines are all important triggers that may induce cellular senescence. Chemotherapy drugs like doxorubicin and cisplatin, for instance, cause cell death and may also induce senescence [85, 86].

As previously mentioned, drug resistance and tumor recurrence/progression might occur as a result of tumor cells evading senescence induced by treatment (TIS) [87]. By acquiring stem-cell characteristics, cancer cells with TIS can avoid senescence and recurrence [88, 89].

1.5 Epigenetic Alterations

Epigenetic changes are an emerging mechanism that contributes to medication resistance. There is growing evidence that epigenetic alterations have a role in the development of resistance mechanisms such as improved drug efflux, accelerated DNA repair, and defective apoptosis [90–93].

DNA methylation, histone modification, chromatin remodeling, and changes to non-coding RNAs are all examples of epigenetic modifications [94]. Increased expression of an oncogene, for instance, would arise from demethylation of DNA in the gene's promoter region, which might lead to resistance to treatment. Recent research showed that in a resistant hepatocellular carcinoma (HCC) cell line, the G-actin monomer binding protein thymosin 4 (T4) was enriched by demethylation of DNA and active modification of histone H3 at the promoter region [95]. The HCC cell line acquired stem cell-like properties with T4 overexpression, and the cells were resistant to the VEGFR inhibitor sorafenib *in vivo* [95].

Non-coding RNAs, including microRNAs (miRNAs) and long non-coding RNAs (lncRNAs), have a significant role in drug resistance [96, 97], in addition to chromosomal alteration. LncRNAs may be anywhere from 200 to over 10,000 nt in length, whereas miRNAs only have approximately 21 to 25 nt. As a result of binding to their corresponding mRNAs, miRNAs mediate mRNA degradation and suppress protein synthesis, earning them a prominent role as regulators of post-transcriptional gene expression. By inhibiting the binding of transcription activators to critical DNA regions in genes and by attracting chromatin remodeling proteins, LncRNAs play a role in the control of gene expression. The expression of proteins involved in cancer medication resistance is controlled by both microRNAs and long noncoding RNAs. It has been demonstrated, for instance, that cisplatin-resistant bladder cancer cells express higher levels of the lncRNA urothelial cancer-associated 1 (UCA1) than susceptible cells [98]. Increasing mRNA and protein levels of wingless-type MMTV integration site family member 6 (Wnt6) was shown to promote Wnt signaling and cell viability when UCA1 expression was upregulated [98].

1.6 Tumor Heterogeneity

Tumors exhibit four types of heterogeneity: genetic, cellular (cancer cells, stromal cells, immune cells, etc.), metabolic (oxygen/nutrient distribution), and temporal (dynamic tumor progression) [99]. Because of tumor heterogeneity, it is almost hard to eradicate all cancer cells with a singular therapy. Combinational therapy, such as FEC (5-fluorouracil, epirubicin, cyclophosphamide) for breast cancer, was developed as a solution to this issue. Here, the authors will discuss about the phenomenon of genetic diversity.

Primary tumors of several cancer types, including ovarian cancer [100], renal cell carcinoma [101], breast cancer [102], and chronic lymphocytic leukemia [103], have been demonstrated to house distinct subpopulations of cancer cells with distinct genetic profiles. Variable clonal variations of a tumor have different sensitivities to chemotherapy and targeted medications, meaning that early treatment can only eradicate some of the tumor while leaving others to persevere. If the resistant clones continue to multiply and expand, the tumor will reappear but this time with a new cell composition that is resistant to the original treatment. Evidence that the subclonal compositions vary dramatically at various periods of therapy [23, 24, 101, 104] lends credence to the idea that genetic heterogeneity of the subpopulations develops during drug treatment in a Darwinian selection way. Exosome-mediated transfer of microRNAs from drug-resistant tumor cells to drug-sensitive tumor cells may cause resistance in both types of tumor cells in heterogeneous tumor cell populations [105].

Studies documenting the decline in responsiveness to targeted medications provide credence to the idea that tumor heterogeneity plays a role in the development of treatment resistance. Targeted medicines have the potential to increase effectiveness and decrease adverse effects, but their high specificity may become a drawback when confronting tumor heterogeneity. Therefore, multi-drug combination therapy is necessary to either prevent tumor recurrence entirely or significantly slow its progression.

And since different individuals may react differently to the same medication, research into customized medicines is critically needed.

1.7 Tumor Microenvironment

Different cell types and the extracellular matrix (ECM) all have a role in the development, progression, and metastasis of tumors [106, 107]. The microenvironment of solid tumors consists of an extracellular matrix (ECM), immunological and inflammatory cells, blood arteries, fibroblasts, and numerous nutrients and signaling chemicals. Together, they play crucial roles in tumor development and survival.

TME has been linked to cancer's innate resistance to treatment. The TME variables include pH. The pH outside of healthy tissue or cell is somewhat higher than the pH inside of it (pHe7.3–7.5 vs. pHi6.8–7.2) [108]. However, cancer cells raise internal pH and decrease external pH by pumping protons through proton transporters and modulating pH sensors [109, 110], creating a so-called reversed pH gradient. According to some research [111], cancer cells' extracellular environment, which is often acidic (pH 6.5–7.1), may contribute to their resistance to chemotherapeutics. Cancer cells are able to avoid apoptosis because the distribution of weak base anticancer medications is hampered by the inverted pH gradient, a phenomenon known as "ion trapping" [112, 113]. The low extracellular pH that is increasingly being seen in solid tumors is a novel signature of these diseases that might be targeted in cancer treatment. Proton pump inhibitors (PPIs) and other therapeutic strategies that aim to lower the acidity of the microenvironment have been developed and proved to be effective in reducing tumor size and making cancer cells more sensitive to chemotherapy. One proton pump inhibitor (PPI) that has been shown to work synergistically with paclitaxel in melanoma cells *in vitro* and *in vivo* is lansoprazole [114].

Adaptation of cancer cells to chemo or targeted treatments, which reduces drug effectiveness and induces resistance, is also facilitated by post-treatment changes in the composition of TME. For instance, in the case of glioblastoma multiforme (GBM), a particularly deadly kind of brain tumor, TAMs contribute to the development of resistance to anticancer therapies [115]. To aid cancer cell growth and survival, macrophages in GBM tumors release large amounts of colony-stimulating factor-1 (CSF-1) [115, 116]. Cancer therapy that employs small molecule inhibitors or antibodies against CSF-1 receptor (CSF-1R) has shown encouraging *in vivo* effects [117–119]. Increased insulin-like growth factor-1 (IGF-1) production from TAMs and IGF-1–induced increase of phosphatidylinositol 3-kinase (PI3K) pathway signaling in glioblastoma multiforme (GBM) tumor cells contribute to the recurrence of GBM in over 50% of patients [115]. It has been shown in animal models that blocking both the CSF-1R and the IGF-1 receptor or PI3K signaling together increases survival time. Therefore, combination treatments that concurrently target cancer cells and TME may result in significantly increased anticancer effectiveness by lowering drug resistance.

Furthermore, TME heterogeneity enriches genetic heterogeneity, which is itself a facet of tumor heterogeneity. Variable hypoxia is one feature of the TME [120], which occurs because tumor vasculature is variable and dynamic. Oxidative stress caused by repeated hypoxia and reoxygenation may cause DNA damage in tumor cells, leading to an increase in mutations and the emergence of genetically distinct clonal subpopulations [121]. Further, as was previously indicated, cells in the TME, such as TAMs, contribute to tumor heterogeneity by interfering with the expression patterns of cancer cells by the release of exosomes carrying miRNAs [38].

As a result, TME is very important in tumor development and resistance to treatment. A more complete understanding of the TME and its interaction with tumor cells might significantly improve therapeutic response and clinical outcomes.

1.8 Epithelial to Mesenchymal Transition

The epithelial-to-mesenchymal transition (EMT) is a process in which epithelial cells change into mesenchymal stem cells by detaching from one another. While it is well established that EMT is necessary for the development of metastasis in cancers of epithelial origin, its involvement in other malignancies, such as sarcomas, is less well understood. There is mounting evidence that EMT is a key player in the development of resistance to chemotherapy. According to research conducted on an EMT lineage-tracing mice model by Fischer *et al.*, EMT enhances resistance to apoptotic induction initiated by the medication cyclophosphamide [122]. Recent research has shown that EMT and CSC have certain commonalities, and their involvements in drug resistance reflect various expressions of the same phenotype; however, the mechanisms of EMT-induced drug resistance are still not well understood. The Wnt, Notch, and Hedgehog signaling pathways are all shared by EMT cells and cancer stem cells (CSCs), suggesting a common mechanism [123]. In this way, EMT provides tumor cells a means to develop resistance to anticancer treatments and avoid the cell death that is normally produced by these medications. Among the best-studied important cytokines in EMT is transforming growth factor beta, whose signaling pathways are linked to acquired drug resistance [124, 125]. Reversing EMT and dramatically increasing cancer cells' susceptibility to chemotherapies have both been linked to TGF- inhibition [126, 127]. Drug resistance has also been linked to the Wnt and Hedgehog pathways, according to the literature [128, 129].

In addition, there is mounting evidence that the EMT program is a crucial regulator of CSCs in mediating drug resistance. Epigenetic alterations triggered by EMT are necessary for cancer cells to enter the CSC state. The field of anticancer therapies would benefit greatly from research into the molecular relationship between EMT, CSCs, and drug resistance [130].

Transcription factors that induce EMT (EMT-TFs) also contribute to the development of drug resistance. Drug resistance may be induced by the overexpression of EMT-TFs [131–135], which include Twist, Snail, Slug, ZEB, and FOXC2. Recent research has shown that mice with pancreatic ductal adenocarcinoma treated with gemcitabine are more sensitive to the treatment and have a higher survival rate when EMT is suppressed by knocking down EMT transcription factors Twist1 or Snail1 [136]. By facilitating

ABC transporter-mediated drug efflux, several of these EMT-TFs contribute to resistance. Binding sites for EMT-TF were identified in the promoters of genes encoding ABC transporters [137]. Through increasing ABCB1 expression and activity, overexpression of Twist, ZEB1/2, Slug, and Snail causes drug resistance [138–140]. It is known that Snail, MSX2, SOX2, and ZEB1 control ABCG2, another ABC transporter intimately associated with MDR [141–144]. EMT-TFs have also been demonstrated to regulate other MDR-related ABC transporters, including ABCC1, ABCC2, ABCC4, and ABCC5. When it comes to paclitaxel-resistant nasopharyngeal cancer cells, for instance, overexpression of ABCC5 is linked to FOXM1. Depletion of FOXM1 or ABCC5 promotes paclitaxel-induced cell death and lowers drug efflux [145–148]. By inhibiting ABC transporters, knocking down these EMT-TFs makes cancer cells more sensitive to chemotherapeutic drugs [142, 143, 148]. Inhibiting metastasis and medication resistance may both be possible by targeting these EMT-TFs.

It is now thought that microRNAs (miRNAs), in addition to EMT-TFs, are critical molecules that connect EMT and ABC transporters [149]. MicroRNAs (miRNAs) are a kind of endogenous RNA consisting of 20–24 nucleotides that may influence the expression of EMT-related genes that belong to the ABC family [149]. The modulation of ABC transporters by microRNAs has been summarized by Haenisch *et al.* [150]. The majority of miRNAs control ABC transporters at post-transcriptional levels by binding sites in the 3′-untranslated region (3′-UTR), although some miRNAs can regulate ABC transporters at transcriptional levels by binding to the gene promoter region [151]. It has been shown that microRNAs (miRNAs) may control not only the expression of ABC transporters but also EMT indicators. MiR-200c, for instance, has been shown to preserve the epithelial phenotype [154] and to negatively regulate EMT by directly targeting 3'-UTR regions of ZEB1 and ZEB2 [152, 153]. Although miR-200c and miR-145 are examples of miRNAs that negatively control ABC transporters and so limit EMT [155], miR-27a is an example of a miRNA that promotes EMT by positively regulating ABC transporters.

An *et al.* outlined the many ways in which miRNAs govern drug resistance, including their roles in modifying apoptosis and autophagy, controlling the metabolism of anti-cancer drugs, affecting therapeutic targets, and influencing DNA repair [156–158]. MiR-134, miR-487b, and miR-655 overexpression increase TGF-induced EMT and treatment resistance to gefitinib in non-small cell lung cancer, according to a recent study [159]. Resistance to EGFR-TKI is induced by this miRNA cluster, which works by directly suppressing MAGI 2, which in turn dampens PTEN function. Acquired resistance to EGFR-TKIs is linked to a loss of PTEN expression

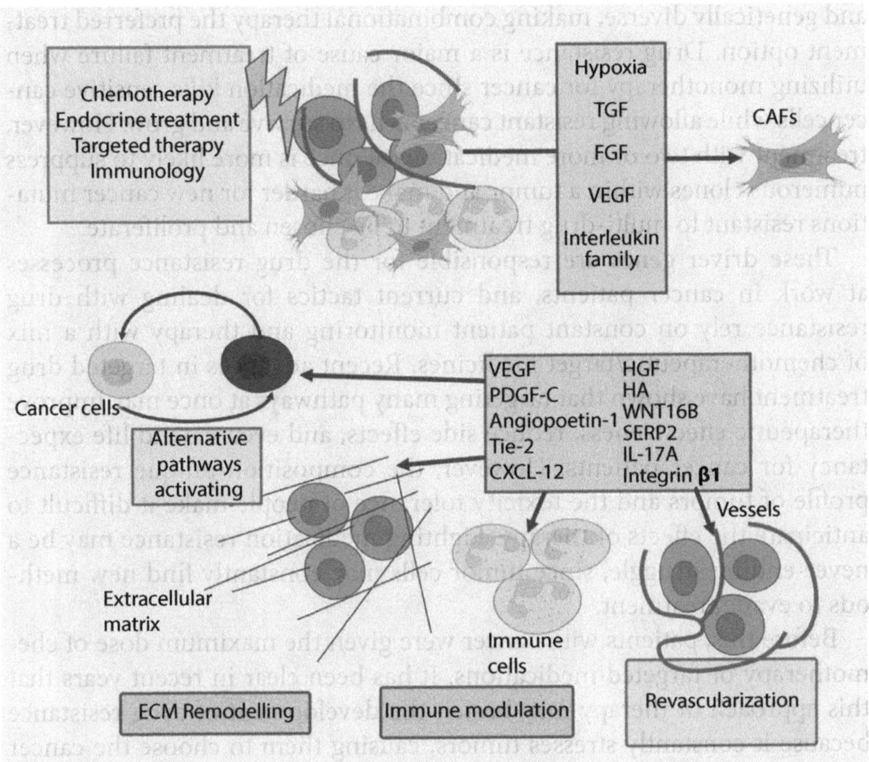

Figure 1.2 Diagrammatic representation of the heterogenous origin of CAFs and their markers.

and an increase in the PI3K–Akt pathway [160]. Heterogeneous origin for CAFs and their marker is shown in Figure 1.2.

1.9 Conclusion

It will be difficult to determine the most effective technique for overcoming medication resistance because of the wide variety of patient malignancies and the intricate nature of tumor growth. High throughput investigations in the fields of cancer genomes, cancer proteomics, and cancer metabolomics have made it feasible to pinpoint the genes and molecules responsible for treatment resistance at any given time during carcinogenesis. Combinational and individualized therapy is necessary because of the heterogeneity of cancer-causing gene alterations. Tumors are often multiclonal and genetically diverse, making combinational therapy the preferred treatment option. Drug resistance is a major cause of treatment failure when utilizing monotherapy for cancer since the medication kills sensitive cancer cells while allowing resistant cancer cells to survive and grow. However, treatment with two or more medications at once is more likely to suppress numerous clones within a tumor and make it harder for new cancer mutations resistant to multi-drug treatment to be chosen and proliferate.

These driver genes are responsible for the drug resistance processes at work in cancer patients, and current tactics for dealing with drug resistance rely on constant patient monitoring and therapy with a mix of chemotherapeutic/target medicines. Recent advances in targeted drug treatment have shown that targeting many pathways at once may improve therapeutic effectiveness, reduce side effects, and even extend life expectancy for cancer patients. However, the composition/unique resistance profile of tumors and the toxicity tolerance of people make it difficult to anticipate the effects of therapy. Fighting medication resistance may be a never-ending struggle, since tumor cells may constantly find new methods to evade treatment.

Before this, patients with cancer were given the maximum dose of chemotherapy or targeted medications. It has been clear in recent years that this approach of therapy may hasten the development of drug resistance because it constantly stresses tumors, causing them to choose the cancer cells that are most resistant to the medications. Intermittent or adaptive dosing may halt the growth of drug-dependent resistant cells and allow for the competition of sensitive and resistant cells, which is why these novel treatment strategies of "on and off" or "high dose followed by low dose" resulted in longer survival and delayed drug resistance. One study demonstrated that melanoma cells that had developed resistance to combination BRAF- and MEK-targeted therapy exhibited classic signs of drug addiction and were highly vulnerable to sudden discontinuation of treatment. The development of drug dependence has been seen in other cancer types as well, such as lymphoma cells exposed to an ALK kinase inhibitor, indicating that intermittent dosing may increase the duration of time in which ALK+ tumors are under control. These results have bolstered the case for clinical trials of a pulsatile dosing strategy.

While some patients saw an increase in survival because of the adoption of novel therapeutic approaches, others saw no improvement or even worse results. These show that the new approaches can only be employed in certain situations and are not applicable as a whole. More research on drug–cancer interactions at the individual level is necessary before tailor-made treatment strategies can be created.

Isolating the source of the tumor's energy might be one way to get around the resistance they have developed. Even if a tumor is able to avoid a certain pathway, it will still require energy to maintain its growth, proliferation, treatment resistance, and cell migration. Therapeutic reagent effectiveness may be enhanced by the use of energy-blocking combinations. Cancer cells, in contrast to normal cells, do not seem to be as adaptable when it comes to utilizing energy molecules. For instance, it is widely established from positron emission tomography (PET) scans that cancers with a poor prognosis are virtually usually tumors with an active glucose/energy metabolism. Glucose is the preferred source of energy and carbon for certain cancer cells. These malignant cells are "addicted" to glucose and are more sensitive to changes in glucose concentration than normal cells, dying at a much quicker rate in the absence of glucose. A combined therapy strategy using a glucose transport inhibitor or a glycolysis inhibitor and another target medicine may be especially useful in triggering cancer cell death in certain specific cancers.

Recent studies on cancer have shown crucial functions for TME in carcinogenesis and treatment resistance. TME–tumor interactions must be taken into account by any novel medicines that aim to considerably enhance therapeutic results. It has become clear that intratumoral extracellular ATP is one of the TME molecules that has significant effects on tumor cells in terms of proliferation, survival, treatment resistance, and even metastasis. While many other molecules may be employed to catalyze the synthesis of ATP, ATP is the final energy molecule utilized by all cells. Increased ATP levels may be essential for the survival and treatment resistance of cancer cells. Understanding this distinction between cancer and healthy cells may aid in the fight against the disease. Deficiencies in ATP might cause tumors to cease growing or even die if a mechanism is discovered and employed to administer an ATP synthesis inhibitor or extracellular ATP degrader, resulting in reduced ATP internalization within tumors. The anticancer efficiency of both TKIs and chemo medicines may be improved by using them in combination treatment, whereby either extracellular ATP destruction or the prevention of extracellular ATP internalization is considered. Since immune cells in tumors are responsive to ATP levels, it is possible that modifying extracellular ATP levels might further improve cancer immunotherapy.

Finally, the heterogeneity of tumor cells should be lower, drug resistance should be lower, and treatment should be more effective if the tumor is found sooner. The relevance of cancer therapy at later stages should not be underestimated, but neither should the importance of early identification and prevention.

References

1. MacConaill, L.E. and Garraway, L.A., Clinical implications of the cancer genome. *J. Clin. Oncol.*, 28, 35, 5219–28, 2010.
2. Goldenberg, M.M., Trastuzumab, a recombinant DNA-derived humanized monoclonal antibody, a novel agent for the treatment of metastatic breast cancer. *Clin. Ther.*, 21, 2, 309–18, 1999.
3. Longley, D.B. and Johnston, P.G., Molecular mechanisms of drug resistance. *J. Pathol.*, 205, 2, 275–92, 2005.
4. Goodman, L.S., Wintrobe, M.M., Dameshek, W., Goodman, M.J., Gilman, A., McLennan, M.T., Nitrogen mustard therapy: Use of methyl-bis (beta-chloroethyl) amine hydrochloride and tris (beta-chloroethyl) amine hydrochloride for hodgkin's disease, lymphosarcoma, leukemia and certain allied and miscellaneous disorders. *JAMA*, 132, 3, 126–32, 1946.
5. Barinaga, M., From bench top to bedside. *Science*, 278, 5340, 1036–9, 1997.
6. Nabholtz, J.M. and Slamon, D., New adjuvant strategies for breast cancer: Meeting the challenge of integrating chemotherapy and trastuzumab (herceptin). *Semin. Oncol.*, 28, 1 Suppl 3, 1–12, 2001.
7. Kreitman, R.J., Immunotoxins for targeted cancer therapy. *AAPS J.*, 8, 3, E532–51, 2006.
8. Benner, S.E., Wahl, G.M., Von Hoff, D.D., Double minute chromosomes and homogeneously staining regions in tumors taken directly from patients versus in human tumor cell lines. *Anticancer Drugs*, 2, 1, 11–25, 1991.
9. Arora, V.K., Schenkein, E., Murali, R., Subudhi, S.K., Wongvipat, J., Balbas, M.D. *et al.*, Glucocorticoid receptor confers resistance to antiandrogens by bypassing androgen receptor blockade. *Cell*, 155, 6, 1309–22, 2013.
10. Gupta, P.B., Fillmore, C.M., Jiang, G., Shapira, S.D., Tao, K., Kuperwasser, C. *et al.*, Stochastic state transitions give rise to phenotypic equilibrium in populations of cancer cells. *Cell*, 146, 4, 633–44, 2011.
11. Kreso, A., O'Brien, C.A., van Galen, P., Gan, O.I., Notta, F., Brown, A.M. *et al.*, Variable clonal repopulation dynamics influence chemotherapy response in colorectal cancer. *Science*, 339, 6119, 543–8, 2013.
12. Nathanson, D.A., Gini, B., Mottahedeh, J., Visnyei, K., Koga, T., Gomez, G. *et al.*, Targeted therapy resistance mediated by dynamic regulation of extrachromosomal mutant EGFR DNA. *Science*, 343, 6166, 72–6, 2014.
13. Gatenby, R.A., Gillies, R.J., Brown, J.S., The evolutionary dynamics of cancer prevention. *Nat. Rev. Cancer*, 10, 8, 526–7, 2010.
14. Junttila, M.R. and de Sauvage, F.J., Influence of tumour micro-environment heterogeneity on therapeutic response. *Nature*, 501, 7467, 346–54, 2013.
15. Li, Z.W. and Dalton, W.S., Tumor microenvironment and drug resistance in hematologic malignancies. *Blood Rev.*, 20, 6, 333–42, 2006.
16. Dalton, W.S., The tumor microenvironment: Focus on myeloma. *Cancer Treat. Rev.*, 29, Suppl 1, 11–9, 2003.

17. Hazlehurst, L.A., Landowski, T.H., Dalton, W.S., Role of the tumor microenvironment in mediating *de novo* resistance to drugs and physiological mediators of cell death. *Oncogene*, 22, 47, 7396–402, 2003.
18. Pal, B., Bayat-Mokhtari, R., Li, H., Bhuyan, R., Talukdar, J., Sandhya, S. *et al.*, Stem cell altruism may serve as a novel drug resistance mechanism in oral cancer. *Cancer Res.*, 76, 14 Supplement, 251, 2016.
19. Settleman, J., Cancer: Bet on drug resistance. *Nature*, 529, 7586, 289–90, 2016.
20. Dean, M., Fojo, T., Bates, S., Tumour stem cells and drug resistance. *Nat. Rev. Cancer*, 5, 4, 275–84, 2005.
21. Druker, B.J., Sawyers, C.L., Kantarjian, H., Resta, D.J., Reese, S.F., Ford, J.M. *et al.*, Activity of a specific inhibitor of the BCR-ABL tyrosine kinase in the blast crisis of chronic myeloid leukemia and acute lymphoblastic leukemia with the philadelphia chromosome. *N. Engl. J. Med.*, 344, 14, 1038–42, 2001.
22. Zahreddine, H. and Borden, K.L., Mechanisms and insights into drug resistance in cancer. *Front. Pharmacol.*, 4, 28, 2013.
23. Michael, M. and Doherty, M.M., Tumoral drug metabolism: Overview and its implications for cancer therapy. *J. Clin. Oncol.*, 23, 1, 205–29, 2005.
24. Sampath, D., Cortes, J., Estrov, Z., Du, M., Shi, Z., Andreeff, M. *et al.*, Pharmacodynamics of cytarabine alone and in combination with 7-hydroxystaurosporine (UCN-01) in AML blasts *in vitro* and during a clinical trial. *Blood*, 107, 6, 2517–24, 2006.
25. Townsend, D.M. and Tew, K.D., The role of glutathione-S-transferase in anti-cancer drug resistance. *Oncogene*, 22, 47, 7369–75, 2003.
26. Manolitsas, T.P., Englefield, P., Eccles, D.M., Campbell, I.G., No association of a 306-bp insertion polymorphism in the progesterone receptor gene with ovarian and breast cancer. *Br. J. Cancer*, 75, 9, 1398–9, 1997.
27. Cumming, R.C., Lightfoot, J., Beard, K., Youssoufian, H., O'Brien, P.J., Buchwald, M., Fanconi anemia group C protein prevents apoptosis in hematopoietic cells through redox regulation of GSTP1. *Nat. Med.*, 7, 7, 814–20, 2001.
28. Juliano, R.L. and Ling, V., A surface glycoprotein modulating drug permeability in chinese hamster ovary cell mutants. *Biochim. Biophys. Acta*, 455, 1, 152–62, 1976.
29. Chen, C.J., Chin, J.E., Ueda, K., Clark, D.P., Pastan, I., Gottesman, M.M. *et al.*, Internal duplication and homology with bacterial transport proteins in the mdr1 (P-glycoprotein) gene from multi-drug-resistant human cells. *Cell*, 47, 3, 381–9, 1986.
30. Croop, J.M., Raymond, M., Haber, D., Devault, A., Arceci, R.J., Gros, P. *et al.*, The three mouse multi-drug resistance (mdr) genes are expressed in a tissue-specific manner in normal mouse tissues. *Mol. Cell Biol.*, 9, 3, 1346–50, 1989.
31. Watson, J.V., *Introduction to flow cytometry*, Cambridge University Press, Cambridge, 2004.

32. Lothstein, L., Hsu, S.I., Horwitz, S.B., Greenberger, L.M., Alternate overexpression of two P-glycoprotein [corrected] genes is associated with changes in multi-drug resistance in a J774.2 cell line. *J. Biol. Chem.*, 264, 27, 16054–8, 1989.
33. Higgins, C.F., ABC transporters: From microorganisms to man. *Annu. Rev. Cell Biol.*, 8, 67–113, 1992.
34. de Vree, J.M., Jacquemin, E., Sturm, E., Cresteil, D., Bosma, P.J., Aten, J. *et al.*, Mutations in the MDR3 gene cause progressive familial intrahepatic cholestasis. *Proc. Natl. Acad. Sci. U. S. A.*, 95, 1, 282–7, 1998.
35. Longo-Sorbello, G.S. and Bertino, J.R., Current understanding of methotrexate pharmacology and efficacy in acute leukemias. *Haematologica*, 86, 2, 121–7, 2001.
36. Inaba, H., Greaves, M., Mullighan, C.G., Acute lymphoblastic leukaemia. *Lancet*, 381, 9881, 1943–55, 2013.
37. Ribera, J.M., Acute lymphoblastic leukemia, in: *HIV-Associated Hematological Malignancies*, M. Hentrich and S. Barta (Eds.), pp. 145–51, Springer, Switzerland, 2016.
38. Jones, D., Kamel-Reid, S., Bahler, D., Dong, H., Elenitoba-Johnson, K., Press, R. *et al.*, Laboratory practice guidelines for detecting and reporting BCR-ABL drug resistance mutations in chronic myelogenous leukemia and acute lymphoblastic leukemia: A report of the Association for Molecular Pathology. *J. Mol. Diagn.*, 11, 1, 4–11, 2009.
39. Simon, J.A. and Kingston, R.E., Occupying chromatin: Polycomb mechanisms for getting to genomic targets, stopping transcriptional traffic, and staying put. *Mol. Cell.*, 49, 5, 808–24, 2013.
40. Housman, G., Byler, S., Heerboth, S., Lapinska, K., Longacre, M., Snyder, N. *et al.*, Drug resistance in cancer: An overview. *Cancers (Basel)*, 6, 3, 1769–92, 2014.
41. Szakas, G., Annereau, J., Lababidi, S., Shankavaram, U., Arciello, A., Bussey, K., Reinhold, W., Guo, Y., Kruh, G., Reimers, M. *et al.*, Predicting drug sensitivity and resistance: Profiling ABC transporter genes in cancer cells. *Cancer Cell*, 6, 129–137, 2004.
42. Hilgendorf, C., Ahlin, G., Seithel, A., Artursson, P., Ungell, A., Karlsson, J., Expression of thirty-six drug transporter genes in human intestine, liver, kidney, and organotypic cell lines. *Drug Metab. Dispos.*, 35, 1333–1340, 2007.
43. Abolhoda, A., Wilson, A., Ross, H., Danenberg, P.V., Burt, M., Scotto, K.W., Rapid activation of MDR1 gene expression in human metastatic sarcoma after *in vivo* exposure to doxorubicin. *Clin. Cancer Res.*, 5, 3352–3356, 1999.
44. Haber, M., Smith, J., Bordow, S., Flemming, C., Cohn, S., London, W., Marshall, G., Norris, M., Association of high-level MRP1 expression with poor clinical outcome in a large prospective study of neuroblastoma. *J. Clin. Oncol.*, 24, 1546–1553, 2006.

45. Yanase, K., Tsukahara, S., Asada, S., Ishikawa, E., Imai, Y., Sugimoto, Y., Gefitinib reverses breast cancer resistance protein-mediated drug resistance. *Mol. Cancer Ther.*, 3, 1119–1125, 2004.
46. Doyle, L.A., Yang, W., Abruzzo, L.V., Krogmann, T., Gao, Y., Rishi, A.K., Ross, D.D., A multi-drug resistance transporter from human MCF-7 breast cancer cells. *Proc. Natl. Acad. Sci. U.S.A.*, 95, 15665–15670, 1998.
47. Imai, Y., Ishikawa, E., Asada, S., Sugimoto, Y., Estrogenmediated post transcriptional down-regulation of breast cancer resistance protein/ABCG2. *Cancer Res.*, 65, 596–604, 2005.
48. Mutoh, K., Tsukahara, S., Mitsuhashi, J., Katayama, K., Sugimoto, Y., Estrogen-mediated post transcriptional downregulation of P-glycoprotein in *MDR1*-transduced human breast cancer cells. *Cancer Sci.*, 97, 1198–1204, 2006.
49. Katayama, K., Yoshioka, S., Tsukahara, S., Mitsuhashi, J., Sugimoto, Y., Inhibition of the mitogen-activated protein kinase pathway results in the down-regulation of P-glycoprotein. *Mol. Cancer Ther.*, 6, 2092–2102, 2007.
50. Fukuyo, Y., Hunt, C.R., Horikoshi, N., Geldanamycinand its anticancer activities. *Cancer Lett.*, 290, 24–35, 2010.
51. Bonanno, L., Favaretto, A., Rosell, R., Platinum drugs and DNA repair mechanism in lung cancer. *Anticancer Res.*, 34, 493–502, 2014.
52. Olaussen, K., Dunant, A., Fouret, P., Brambilla, E., Andre, F., Haddad, V., Taranchon, E., Filipits, M., Pirker, R., Helmut, P. *et al.*, DNA repair by ERCC1 in non-small-cell lung cancer and cisplatin-based adjuvant chemotherapy. *N. Engl. J. Med.*, 355, 983–991, 2006.
53. Selvakumaran, M., Pisarcik, D., Bao, R., Yeung, A., Hamilton, T., Enhanced cisplatin cytotoxicity by disturbing the nucleotide excision repair pathway in ovarian cancer cell lines. *Cancer Res.*, 63, 1311–1316, 2003.
54. Curtin, N.J., DNA repair dysregulation from cancer driver to therapeutic target. *Nat. Rev.*, 12, 801–817, 2012.
55. Esteller, M., Epigenetic lesions causing genetic lesions in human cancer: Promoter hypermethylation of DNA repair genes. *Eur. J. Cancer*, 36, 2294–2300, 2000.
56. Goode, E., Ulrich, C., Potter, J., Polymorphisms in DNA repair genes and associations with cancer risk. *Cancer Epidemiol. Biomarkers Prev.*, 11, 1513–1530, 2002.
57. Maier, P., Spier, I., Laufs, S., Veldwijk, M.R., Fruehauf, S., Wenz, F., Zeller, W.J., Chemoprotection of human hematopoietic stem cells by simultaneous lentiviral overexpression of multi-drug resistance 1 and O(6)-methylguanine-DNA methyltransferase(P140K). *Gene Ther.*, 17, 389–399, 2010.
58. Blanc, J.L., Wager, M., Guilhot, J., Kusy, S., Bataille, B., Chantereau, T., Lapierre, F., Larsen, C.J., Karayan-Tapon, L., Correlation of clinical features and methylation status of MGMT gene promoter in glioblastomas. *J. Neurooncol.*, 68, 275–283, 2004.

59. Rabik, C., Fishel, M., Holleran, J., Kasza, K., Kelley, M., Egorin, M., Dolan, M., Enhancement of cisplatin cytotoxicity by O6-benzylguanine involves endoplasmic reticulum stress. *J. Pharmacol. Exp. Ther.*, 327, 442–452, 2008.
60. Gegi, M., Diserens, A., Gorlia, T., Hamou, M., de Tribolet, N., Weller, M., Kros, J., Hainfellner, J., Mason, W., Mariani, L. *et al.*, MGMT gene silencing and benefit from temozolomide in glioblastoma. *N. Engl. J. Med.*, 352, 997–1003, 2005.
61. Dong, X., Liu, R., Chen, W., Correlation of promoter methylation in MGMT gene with glioma risk and prognosis: A meta-analysis. *Mol. Neurobiol.*, 52, 1–2, 2014.
62. Frew, A.J., Lindemann, R.K., Martin, B.P., Combination therapy of established cancer using a histone deacetylase inhibitor and a TRAIL receptor agonist. *Proc. Natl. Acad. Sci. U.S.A.*, 105, 11317–11322, 2008.
63. Soria, J., Smit, E., Khayat, D., Besse, B., Yang, X., Hsu, C., Reese, D., Wiezorek, J., Blackhall, F., Phase 1b study of dulanermin (recombinant human Apo2L/TRAIL) in combination with paclitaxel, carboplatin, and bevacizumanb in patients with advanced non-squamous non-small-cell lung cancer. *J. Clin. Oncol.*, 28, 1527–1533, 2010.
64. Mataga, M., Rosenthal, S., Heerboth, S., Devalapalli, A., Kokolus, S., Evans, L.R., Longacre, M., Housman, G., Sarkar, S., Anti-breast cancer effects of histone deacetylase inhibitors and calpain inhibitors. *Anticancer Res.*, 32, 2523–2530, 2012.
65. Sarkar, S. and Faller, D.V., T-oligos inhibit growth and induce apoptosis in human ovarian cancer cells. *Oligonucleoties*, 21, 47–53, 2011.
66. Sarkar, S. and Faller, D.V., Telomere-homilogous G-rich oligonucleotides sensitize human ovarian cancer cells by combination therapy. *Nucleic Acid Ther.*, 23, 167–174, 2013.
67. Sasaki, K., Tsuno, N.H., Sunami, E., Tsurita, G., Kawai, K., Okaji, Y., Nishikawa, T., Shuno, Y., Hongo, K., Hiyoshi, M. *et al.*, Chloroquine potentiates the anticancer effect of 5-fluorouracil on colon cancer cells. *BMC Cancer*, 10, e370, 2010.
68. Cook, K.L., Wärri, A., Soto-Pantoja, D.R., Clarke, P.A.G., Cruz, M.I., Zwart, A., Clarke, R., Hydroxychloroquine inhibits autophagy to potentiate antiestrogen responsiveness in ER+ breast cancer. *Clin. Cancer Res.*, 20, 3222–3232, 2014.
69. Shang, Y., Cai, X., Fan, D., Roles of epithelial-mesenchymal transition in cancer drug resistance. *Curr. Cancer Drug Targets*, 13, 915–929, 2013.
70. Singh, A. and Settleman J., E.M.T., cancer stem cells and drug resistance: An emerging axis of evil in the war on cancer. *Oncogene*, 29, 4741–4751, 2010.
71. Chaffer, C., Brueckmann, I., Scheel, C., Kaestli, A., Wiggins, P., Rodrigues, L., Brooks, M., Reinhardt, F., Su, Y., Polyak, K. *et al.*, Normal and neoplastic nonstem cells can spontaneously covert to a stem-like state. *Proc. Natl. Acad. Sci. U.S.A.*, 108, 7950–7955, 2011.

72. Chaffer, C. and Weinberg R., A perspective on cancer cell metastasis. *Science*, 331, 1559–1564, 2011.
73. Sarkar, S., Horn, G., Moulton, K., Oza, A., Byler, S., Kokolus, S., Longacre, M., Cancer development, progression and therapy: An epigenetic overview. *Int. J. Mol. Sci.*, 14, 21087–21113, 2013.
74. Byler, S., Goldgar, S., Heerboth, S., Leary, M., Housman, G., Moulton, K., Sarkar, S., Genetic and epigenetic aspects of breast cancer progression and therapy. *Anticancer Res.*, 34, 1071–1077, 2014.
75. Li, J.H., Luo, N., Zhong, M.Z., Xiao, Z.Q., Wang, J.X., Yao, X.Y. *et al.*, Inhibition of MicroRNA-196a might reverse cisplatin resistance of A549/DDP non-small-cell lung cancer cell line. *Tumor Biol.*, 37, 2, 2387–94, 2016.
76. Sui, H., Cai, G.X., Pan, S.F., Deng, W.L., Wang, Y.W., Chen, Z.S. *et al.*, miR200c attenuates P-gp-mediated MDR and metastasis by targeting JNK2/c-Jun signaling pathway in colorectal cancer. *Mol. Cancer Ther.*, 13, 12, 3137–51, 2014.
77. Shen, X., Guo, Y., Qi, J., Shi, W., Wu, X., Ni, H. *et al.*, Study on the association between miRNA-202 expression and drug sensitivity in multiple myeloma cells. *Pathol. Oncol. Res.*, 22, 3, 531–9, 2016.
78. Zhang, A.X., Lu, F.Q., Yang, Y.P., Ren, X.Y., Li, Z.F., Zhang, W., MicroRNA-217 overexpression induces drug resistance and invasion of breast cancer cells by targeting PTEN signaling. *Cell Biol. Int.*, 42, 1–10, 2015.
79. Gullà, A., Di Martino, M.T., Gallo Cantafio, M.E., Morelli, E., Amodio, N., Botta, C. *et al.*, A 13 mer LNA-i-miR-221 inhibitor restores drug sensitivity in melphalan-refractory multiple myeloma cells. *Clin. Cancer Res.*, 22, 5, 1222–33, 2016.
80. Shang, Y., Zhang, Z., Liu, Z., Feng, B., Ren, G., Li, K. *et al.*, miR-508-5p regulates multi-drug resistance of gastric cancer by targeting ABCB1 and ZNRD1. *Oncogene*, 33, 25, 3267–76, 2014.
81. To, K.K., Leung, W.W., Ng, S.S., Exploiting a novel miR-519c-HuR-ABCG2 regulatory pathway to overcome chemoresistance in colorectal cancer. *Exp. Cell Res.*, 338, 2, 222–31, 2015.
82. van Jaarsveld, M.T., van Kuijk, P.F., Boersma, A.W., Helleman, J., van, I.W.F., Mathijssen, R.H. *et al.*, miR-634 restores drug sensitivity in resistant ovarian cancer cells by targeting the Ras-MAPK pathway. *Mol. Cancer*, 14, 196, 2015.
83. Hiraki, M., Nishimura, J., Takahashi, H., Wu, X., Takahashi, Y., Miyo, M. *et al.*, Concurrent targeting of KRAS and AKT by MiR-4689 is a novel treatment against mutant KRAS colorectal cancer. *Mol. Ther. Nucleic Acids*, 4, e231, 2015.
84. Mansoori, B., Mohammadi, A., Shirjang, S., Baradaran, B., Micro-RNAs: The new potential biomarkers in cancer diagnosis, prognosis and cancer therapy. *Cell. Mol. Biol. (Noisy-le-Grand)*, 61, 5, 1–10, 2015.
85. Montazami, N., Kheir Andish, M., Majidi, J., Yousefi, M., Yousefi, B., Mohamadnejad, L. *et al.*, siRNA-mediated silencing of MDR1 reverses the

resistance to oxaliplatin in SW480/OxR colon cancer cells. *Cell. Mol. Biol. (Noisy-le-Grand)*, 61, 2, 98–103, 2015.

86. Mansoori, B., Mohammadi, A., Goldar, S., Shanehbandi, D., Mohammadnejad, L., Baghbani, E. *et al.*, Silencing of high mobility group isoform I-C (HMGI-C) enhances paclitaxel chemosensitivity in breast adenocarcinoma cells (MDA-MB-468). *Adv. Pharm. Bull.*, 6, 2, 171–7, 2016.
87. Kachalaki, S., Baradaran, B., Majidi, J., Yousefi, M., Shanehbandi, D., Mohammadinejad, S. *et al.*, Reversal of chemoresistance with small interference RNA (siRNA) in etoposide resistant acute myeloid leukemia cells (HL-60). *Biomed. Pharmacother.*, 75, 100–4, 2015.
88. Mansoori, B., Sandoghchian Shotorbani, S., Baradaran, B., RNA interference and its role in cancer therapy. *Adv. Pharm. Bull.*, 4, 4, 313–21, 2014.
89. Ning, Y., Gerger, A., Zhang, W., Hanna, D.L., Yang, D., Winder, T., Wakatsuki, T., Labonte, M.J., Stintzing, S., Volz, N. *et al.*, Plastin polymorphisms predict gender- and stage-specific colon cancer recurrence after adjuvant chemotherapy. *Mol. Cancer Ther.*, 13, 528–539, 2014.
90. Bégué, E., Jean-Louis, F., Bagot, M., Jauliac, S., Cayuela, J.M., Laroche, L., Parquet, N., Bachelez, H., Bensussan, A., Courtois, G. *et al.*, Inducible expression and pathophysiologic functions of T-plastin in cutaneous T-cell lymphoma. *Blood*, 120, 143–154, 2012.
91. Staussman, R., Morikawa, T., Shee, K., Barzily-Rokni, M., Qian, Z.R., Du, J., Davis, A., Mongare, M.M., Gould, J., Frederick, D.T. *et al.*, Tumor microenvironment elicits innate resistance to RAF inhibitors through HGF secretion. *Nature*, 487, 500–504, 2012.
92. Parkin, B., Ouillette, P., Li, Y., Keller, J., Lam, C., Roulston, D., Li, C., Shedden, K., Malek, S.N., Clonal evolution and devolution after chemotherapy in adult acute myelogenous leukemia. *Blood*, 121, 369–377, 2013.
93. Navin, N., Krasnitz, A., Rodgers, L., Cook, K., Meth, J., Kendall, J., Riggs, M., Eberling, Y., Troge, J., Grubor, V. *et al.*, Inferring tumor progression from genomic heterogeneity. *Genome Res.*, 20, 68–80, 2010.
94. Campbell, P., Yachida, S., Mudie, L., Stephens, P., Pleasance, E., Stebbings, L., Morsberger, L., Latimer, C., McLaren, S., Lin, M. *et al.*, The patterns and dynamics of genomic instability in metastatic pancreatic cancer. *Nature*, 467, 1109–1113, 2010.
95. Baker, E.K. and El-Osta, A., The rise of DNA methylation and the importance of chromatin on multi-drug resistance in cancer. *Exp. Cell Res.*, 290, 177–194, 2003.
96. Kantharidis, P., El-Oska, A., de Silva, M., Wall, D.M., Hu, X.F., Slater, A., Nadalin, G., Parkin, J.D., Zalcberg, J.R., Altered methylation of the human MDR1 promoter is associated with acquired multi-drug resistance. *Clin. Cancer Res.*, 3, 2025–2032, 1997.
97. Plumb, J.A., Strathdee, G., Sludden, J., Kaye, S.B., Brown, R., Reversal of drug resistance in human tumor xenografts by 2'-deoxy-5-azacytidine-induced

demethylation of the hMLH1 gene promoter. *Cancer Res.*, 60, 6039–6044, 2000.
98. Arnold, C.N., Goel, A., Boland, C.R., Role of MLH1 promoter hypermethylation in drug resistance to 5-flurouracil in colorectal cancer cell lines. *Int. J. Cancer*, 106, 66–73, 2003.
99. Bearzatto, A., Szadkowski, M., Macpherson, P., Jiricny, J., Karran, P., Epigenetic regulation of the MGMT and hMSH6 DNA repair genes in cells resistant to methylating agents. *Cancer Res.*, 60, 3262–3270, 2000.
100. Esteller, M., Garcia-Foncillas, J., Andion, E., Goodman, S.N., Hidalgo, O.F., Vanaclocha, V., Baylin, S.B., Herman, J.G., Inactivation of DNA-repair gene MGMT and the clinical response of gliomas to alkylating agents. *N. Engl. J. Med.*, 343, 1350–1354, 2000.
101. Worm, J., Kirkin, A.F., Dzhandzhugazyan, K.N., Guldberg, P., Methylation-dependent silencing of the reduced folate carrier gene in inherently methotrexate-resistant human breast cancer cells. *J. Biol. Chem.*, 276, 39990–40000, 2001.
102. Chang, H.G., Kim, S.J., Chung, K.W., Noh, D.Y., Kwon, Y., Lee, E.S., Kang, H.S., Tamoxifen-resistant breast cancer show less frequent methylation of the estrogen receptor beta but not the estrogen receptor alpha gene. *J. Mol. Med.*, 83, 132–139, 2005.
103. Christmann, M., Pick, M., Lage, H., Schadendorf, D., Kaina, B., Acquired resistance of melanoma cells to the antineoplastic agent fotemustine is caused by reactivation of the DNA repair gene MGMT. *Int. J. Cancer*, 92, 123–129, 2001.
104. Izbicka, E., MacDonald, J.R., Davidson, K., Lawrence, R.A., Gomez, L., von Hoff, D.D., 5,6 Dihydro-5'-azacytidine (DHAC) restores androgen responsiveness in androgen-insensitive prostate cancer cells. *Anticancer Res.*, 19, 1285–1291, 1999.
105. Sarkar, S., Abujamra, A.L., Loew, J.E., Forman, L.W., Perrine, S.P., Faller, D.V., Histone deacetylase inhibitors reverse CpG methylation by regulating DNMT1 through ERK signaling. *Anticancer Res.*, 31, 2723–2732, 2011.
106. Housman, G., Mataga, A.M., Devalapalli, A., Heerboth, S., Evans, L.R., Sarkar, S., Demethylation and re-expression of tumor suppressor genes by HDAC inhibitors and calpain inhibitors in cancer cells: A study related to synergistic type growth inhibition and reduction of motility. *The Epigenetics World Congress*, MA, USA, April 2011, Abstract 206.
107. Sarkar, S., Goldgar, S., Byler, S., Rosenthal, S., Heerboth, S., Demethylation and re-expression of epigenetically silenced tumor suppressor genes: Sensitization of cancer cells by combination therapy. *Epigenomics*, 5, 87–94, 2013.
108. Juergens, R., Wrangle, J., Vendetti, F., Murphy, S.C., Zhao, M., Coleman, B., Sebree, R., Rodgers, K., Hooker, C.M., Franco, N. *et al.*, Combination epigenetic therapy has efficacy in patients with refractory advanced non-small cell lung cancer. *Cancer Discovery*, 1, 598–607, 2011.

109. Johannessen, C.M., Johnson, L.A., Piccioni, F., Townes, A., Frederick, D.T., Donahue, M.K., Narayan, R., Flaherty, K.T., Wargo, J.A., Root, D.E. *et al.*, A melanocyte lineage program confers resistance to MAP kinase pathway inhibition. *Nature*, 504, 138–142, 2013.
110. Cacan, E., Ali, M.W., Boyd, N.H., Hooks, S.B., Greer, S.F., Inhibition of HDAC1 and DNMT1 modulate RGS10 expression and decrease ovarian cancer chemoresistance. *PLoS One*, 9, e87455, 2014.
111. Sarkar, S., Longacre, M., Tatur, N., Heerboth, S., Lapinska, K., Histone deacetylases (HDACs): Function, mechanism, & inhibition, in: *Encyclopedia of Analytical Chemistry*, R.A. Meyers (Ed.), pp. 1–9, John Wiley, Chichester, UK, 2014.
112. Heerboth, S., Lapinska, K., Snyder, N., Leary, M., Rollinson, S., Sarkar, S., The use of epigenetic drugs in diseases: An overview. *Genet. Epigenet.*, 6, 9–19, 2014.
113. Gatenby, R.A., Gillies, R.J., Brown, J.S., The evolutionary dynamics of cancer prevention. *Nat. Rev. Cancer*, 10, 8, 526–7, 2010.
114. Junttila, M.R. and de Sauvage, F.J., Influence of tumour micro-environment heterogeneity on therapeutic response. *Nature*, 501, 7467, 346–54, 2013.
115. Li, Z.W. and Dalton, W.S., Tumor microenvironment and drug resistance in hematologic malignancies. *Blood Rev.*, 20, 6, 333–42, 2006.
116. Dalton, W.S., The tumor microenvironment: Focus on myeloma. *Cancer Treat. Rev.*, 29, Suppl 1, 11–9, 2003.
117. Hazlehurst, L.A., Landowski, T.H., Dalton, W.S., Role of the tumor microenvironment in mediating de novo resistance to drugs and physiological mediators of cell death. *Oncogene*, 22, 47, 7396–402, 2003.
118. Pal, B., Bayat-Mokhtari, R., Li, H., Bhuyan, R., Talukdar, J., Sandhya, S. *et al.*, Stem cell altruism may serve as a novel drug resistance mechanism in oral cancer. *Cancer Res.*, 76, 14 Supplement, 251, 2016.
119. Settleman, J., Cancer: Bet on drug resistance. *Nature*, 529, 7586, 289–90, 2016.
120. Dean, M., Fojo, T., Bates, S., Tumour stem cells and drug resistance. *Nat. Rev. Cancer*, 5, 4, 275–84, 2005.
121. Druker, B.J., Sawyers, C.L., Kantarjian, H., Resta, D.J., Reese, S.F., Ford, J.M. *et al.*, Activity of a specific inhibitor of the BCR-ABL tyrosine kinase in the blast crisis of chronic myeloid leukemia and acute lymphoblastic leukemia with the philadelphia chromosome. *N. Engl. J. Med.*, 344, 14, 1038–42, 2001.
122. Zahreddine, H. and Borden, K.L., Mechanisms and insights into drug resistance in cancer. *Front. Pharmacol.*, 4, 28, 2013, doi: 10.3389/fphar.2013.00028.
123. Michael, M. and Doherty, M.M., Tumoral drug metabolism: Overview and its implications for cancer therapy. *J. Clin. Oncol.*, 23, 1, 205–29, 2005.
124. Sampath, D., Cortes, J., Estrov, Z., Du, M., Shi, Z., Andreeff, M. *et al.*, Pharmacodynamics of cytarabine alone and in combination with 7-hydroxystaurosporine (UCN-01) in AML blasts *in vitro* and during a clinical trial. *Blood*, 107, 6, 2517–24, 2006.

125. Townsend, D.M. and Tew, K.D., The role of glutathione-S-transferase in anti-cancer drug resistance. *Oncogene*, 22, 47, 7369–75, 2003.
126. Manolitsas, T.P., Englefield, P., Eccles, D.M., Campbell, I.G., No association of a 306-bp insertion polymorphism in the progesterone receptor gene with ovarian and breast cancer. *Br. J. Cancer*, 75, 9, 1398–9, 1997.
127. Cumming, R.C., Lightfoot, J., Beard, K., Youssoufian, H., O'Brien, P.J., Buchwald, M., Fanconi anemia group C protein prevents apoptosis in hematopoietic cells through redox regulation of GSTP1. *Nat. Med.*, 7, 7, 814–20, 2001.
128. Juliano, R.L. and Ling, V., A surface glycoprotein modulating drug permeability in chinese hamster ovary cell mutants. *Biochim. Biophys. Acta*, 455, 1, 152–62, 1976.
129. Chen, C.J., Chin, J.E., Ueda, K., Clark, D.P., Pastan, I., Gottesman, M.M. *et al.*, Internal duplication and homology with bacterial transport proteins in the mdr1 (P-glycoprotein) gene from multi-drug-resistant human cells. *Cell*, 47, 3, 381–9, 1986.
130. Croop, J.M., Raymond, M., Haber, D., Devault, A., Arceci, R.J., Gros, P. *et al.*, The three mouse multi-drug resistance (mdr) genes are expressed in a tissue-specific manner in normal mouse tissues. *Mol. Cell. Biol.*, 9, 3, 1346–50, 1989.
131. Watson, J.V., *Introduction to flow cytometry*, Cambridge University Press, Cambridge, 2004.
132. Lothstein, L., Hsu, S.I., Horwitz, S.B., Greenberger, L.M., Alternate overexpression of two P-glycoprotein [corrected] genes is associated with changes in multi-drug resistance in a J774.2 cell line. *J. Biol. Chem.*, 264, 27, 16054–8, 1989.
133. Higgins, C.F., ABC transporters: From microorganisms to man. *Annu. Rev. Cell Biol.*, 8, 67–113, 1992.
134. de Vree, J.M., Jacquemin, E., Sturm, E., Cresteil, D., Bosma, P.J., Aten, J. *et al.*, Mutations in the MDR3 gene cause progressive familial intrahepatic cholestasis. *Proc. Natl. Acad. Sci. U. S. A.*, 95, 1, 282–7, 1998.
135. Longo-Sorbello, G.S. and Bertino, J.R., Current understanding of methotrexate pharmacology and efficacy in acute leukemias. *Haematologica*, 86, 2, 121–7, 2001.
136. Inaba, H., Greaves, M., Mullighan, C.G., Acute lymphoblastic leukaemia. *Lancet*, 381, 9881, 1943–55, 2013, doi: 10.1016/S0140-6736(12)62187-4.
137. Ribera, J.M., Acute lymphoblastic leukemia, in: *HIV-Associated Hematological Malignancies*, M. Hentrich and S. Barta (Eds.), pp. 145–51, Springer, Switzerland, 2016.
138. Jones, D., Kamel-Reid, S., Bahler, D., Dong, H., Elenitoba-Johnson, K., Press, R. *et al.*, Laboratory practice guidelines for detecting and reporting BCR-ABL drug resistance mutations in chronic myelogenous leukemia and acute lymphoblastic leukemia: A report of the Association for Molecular Pathology. *J. Mol. Diagn.*, 11, 1, 4–11, 2009.

139. Simon, J.A. and Kingston, R.E., Occupying chromatin: Polycomb mechanisms for getting to genomic targets, stopping transcriptional traffic, and staying put. *Mol. Cell.*, 49, 5, 808–24, 2013.
140. Housman, G., Byler, S., Heerboth, S., Lapinska, K., Longacre, M., Snyder, N. *et al.*, Drug resistance in cancer: An overview. *Cancers (Basel)*, 6, 3, 1769–92, 2014.
141. LaFave, L.M. and Levine, R.L., JAK2 the future: Therapeutic strategies for JAK-dependent malignancies. *Trends Pharmacol. Sci.*, 33, 11, 574–82, 2012.
142. De Toni, F., Racaud-Sultan, C., Chicanne, G., Mas, V.M., Cariven, C., Mesange, F. *et al.*, A crosstalk between the Wnt and the adhesion-dependent signaling pathways governs the chemosensitivity of acute myeloid leukemia. *Oncogene*, 25, 22, 3113–22, 2006.
143. Grandage, V.L., Gale, R.E., Linch, D.C., Khwaja, A., PI3-kinase/Akt is constitutively active in primary acute myeloid leukaemia cells and regulates survival and chemoresistance via NF-kappaB, mapkinase and p53 pathways. *Leukemia*, 19, 4, 586–94, 2005.
144. Luo, J.M., Yoshida, H., Komura, S., Ohishi, N., Pan, L., Shigeno, K. *et al.*, Possible dominant-negative mutation of the SHIP gene in acute myeloid leukemia. *Leukemia*, 17, 1, 1–8, 2003.
145. Hollestelle, A., Elstrodt, F., Nagel, J.H., Kallemeijn, W.W., Schutte, M., Phosphatidylinositol-3-OH kinase or RAS pathway mutations in human breast cancer cell lines. *Mol. Cancer Res.*, 5, 2, 195–201, 2007.
146. Steelman, L.S., Abrams, S.L., Whelan, J., Bertrand, F.E., Ludwig, D.E., Bäsecke, J. *et al.*, Contributions of the Raf/MEK/ERK, PI3K/PTEN/Akt/mTOR and Jak/STAT pathways to leukemia. *Leukemia*, 22, 4, 686–707, 2008.
147. Kim, D., Dan, H.C., Park, S., Yang, L., Liu, Q., Kaneko, S. *et al.*, AKT/PKB signaling mechanisms in cancer and chemoresistance. *Front. Biosci.*, 10, 975–87, 2005.
148. Brown, R., Curry, E., Magnani, L., Wilhelm-Benartzi, C.S., Borley, J., Poised epigenetic states and acquired drug resistance in cancer. *Nat. Rev. Cancer*, 14, 11, 747–53, 2014.
149. Byler, S., Goldgar, S., Heerboth, S., Leary, M., Housman, G., Moulton, K. *et al.*, Genetic and epigenetic aspects of breast cancer progression and therapy. *Anticancer Res.*, 34, 3, 1071–7, 2014.
150. Holohan, C., Van Schaeybroeck, S., Longley, D.B., Johnston, P.G., Cancer drug resistance: An evolving paradigm. *Nat. Rev. Cancer*, 13, 10, 714–26, 2013.
151. Borst, P., Evers, R., Kool, M., Wijnholds, J., A family of drug transporters: The multi-drug resistance-associated proteins. *J. Natl. Cancer Inst.*, 92, 16, 1295–302, 2000.
152. de Pagter, M.S. and Kloosterman, W.P., The diverse effects of complex chromosome rearrangements and chromothripsis in cancer development, in: *Chromosomal Instability in Cancer Cells*, B. Ghadimi and T. Ried (Eds.), pp. 165–93, Springer, Switzerland, 2015.

153. Beach, L.R. and Palmiter, R.D., Amplification of the metallothionein-I gene in cadmium-resistant mouse cells. *Proc. Natl. Acad. Sci. U. S. A.*, 78, 4, 2110–4, 1981.
154. Woolley, P.V. and Tew, K.D., *Mechanisms of drug resistance in neoplastic cells: Bristol-Myers cancer symposia*, Academic Press, Inc., New York, 2013.
155. Matsui, A., Ihara, T., Suda, H., Mikami, H., Semba, K., Gene amplification: Mechanisms and involvement in cancer. *Biomol. Concepts*, 4, 6, 567–82, 2013.
156. Dimude, J.U., Stockum, A., Midgley-Smith, S.L., Upton, A.L., Foster, H.A., Khan, A. *et al.*, The consequences of replicating in the wrong orientation: Bacterial chromosome duplication without an active replication origin. *MBio*, 6, 6, e01294–15, 2015.
157. García-Pérez, J., López-Abente, G., Gómez-Barroso, D., Morales-Piga, A., Romaguera, E.P., Tamayo, I. *et al.*, Childhood leukemia and residential proximity to industrial and urban sites. *Environ. Res.*, 140, 542–53, 2015.
158. Pui, C.H., Yang, J.J., Hunger, S.P., Pieters, R., Schrappe, M., Biondi, A. *et al.*, Childhood acute lymphoblastic leukemia: Progress through collaboration. *J. Clin. Oncol.*, 33, 27, 2938–48, 2015.
159. Baguley, B.C., Classical and targeted anticancer drugs: An appraisal of mechanisms of multi-drug resistance, in: *Cancer Drug Resistance: Methods in Molecular Biology*, J. Rueff and A. Rodrigues (Eds.), pp. 19–37, Humana Press, New York, 2016.
160. Wojtuszkiewicz, A., Assaraf, Y.G., Hoekstra, M., Jansen, G., Peters, G.J., Sonneveld, E. *et al.*, The relevance of aberrant FPGS splicing for *ex vivo* MTX resistance and clinical outcome in childhood acute lymphoblastic leukemia. *Cancer Res.*, 75, 15 Suppl, 4437, 2015.

2

Understanding Different Mechanisms Involved in Cancer Drug Resistance: Proposing Novel Strategies to Overcome MDR

Rishabha Malviya*, Arun Kumar Singh and Deepika Yadav

Abstract
Resistance to anticancer drugs rises when their targets shift. DNA microarray, proteomics, and the development of personalized medicines are all providing novel means of overcoming drug resistance. There has been a rise in the number of novel chemotherapies, but no one has yet succeeded in creating an effective chemotherapeutic agent against advanced cancer (such as invasion and metastasis). Tumor somatic cell genetic variations and other environmental factors may both contribute to cancer cells' resistance to anticancer drugs. Therefore, cancer treatment resistance may be developed via a number of mechanisms, such as decreased apoptosis, altered drug metabolism, altered epigenetics, therapeutic targets, and increased DNA repair. This chapter covered the reasons why cancer medications fail to work and why conventional chemotherapeutics fail to treat cancer.

***Keywords*:** Cancer, multi-drug resistance, microRNA, epigenetic, cell death inhibiting

2.1 Introduction

There are constant shifts in our fundamental understanding of cancer as new findings are discovered in the field. Cancer is defined by its hallmarks, which include the unregulated proliferation of aberrant cells and the dynamic modification of the DNA (which causes malignant traits in normal cells) [1]. The normal metabolic process of healthy cells is

**Corresponding author*: rishabhamalviya19@gmail.com

Rishabha Malviya, Arun Kumar Singh and Deepika Yadav. Multi-Drug Resistance in Cancer: Mechanism and Treatment Strategies, (31–46) © 2023 Scrivener Publishing LLC

disrupted due to the invasion of local tissues and metastasis to distant organs [2].

Other than conventional chemotherapy medications including surgery, radiation treatment, chemotherapy, combination therapy, and laser therapy, selective therapies are based on a deeper understanding of the biology and molecular genetics involved in tumor growth [3].

Despite considerable advances, chemotherapy remains the gold standard for cancer treatment. Invasive and metastatic cancer now accounts for 90 % of treatment failures. Some of the tumor cells develop resistance to the chemotherapy after it has been given to the patient. Accordingly, drug resistance appears to be a major problem in the field of cancer [4]. Resistance to cytotoxic medications and the negative effects of chemotherapy are two of the many problems in cancer treatment [5]. Molecular targets for prospective cancer therapeutics include oncogenes, tumor suppressor genes, and RNA interference (RNAi) [6]. These therapies aim to lessen the large variety of side effects associated with anti-cancer treatments by, among other things, focusing on kinases implicated in cell proliferation and enhancing cancer's responsiveness to the immune system [7]. Drug inactivation, multi-drug resistance, control of cell death (apoptosis suppression), changes in drug metabolism, epigenetic modifications, and pharmacological targets are all factors in chemotherapy resistance (Figure 2.1).

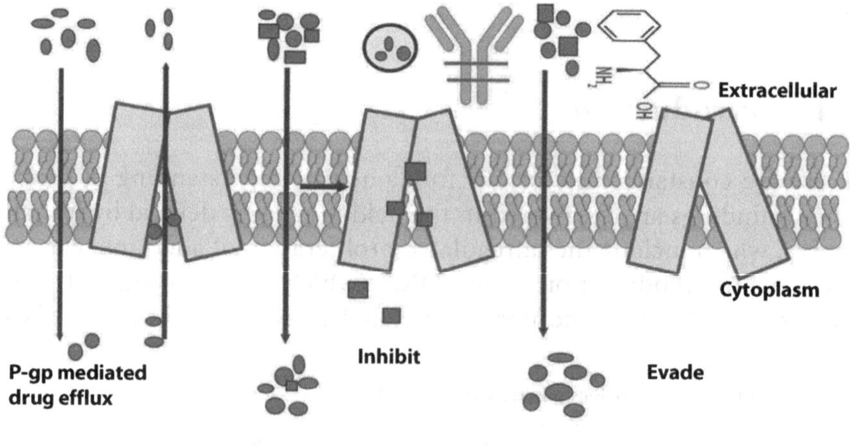

Figure 2.1 The drug release mechanism via the ABC channel outside the cell.

2.2 Drug Resistance: Internal and External Variables

2.2.1 Phenotypic Variation of Tumors

Depending on the stage of cancer, various biological factors may be responsible for the observed intra-tumor heterogeneity. This indicates that many different factors, including those at the genomic, epigenetic, transcriptomic, and proteomic levels, contribute to the development of natural variation. Gene duplications, deletions, and even microRNA (and other small RNA) translocations are all examples of genome changes. Due to chromosomal instability, cancer cells have a high level of intercellular genetic heterogeneity. Increased miRNA, transcriptome, and proteome diversity due to basic genotypic modifications may potentially reflect cell cycle phase, stochastic differences in version between cells, or a hierarchical cell organization in keeping with the cancer stem cell hypothesis [8–12]. In tumors, these factors are referred to as "intrinsic variables." Hypoxia, changes in pH, and paracrine signaling between stromal and other tumor cells are all instances of extrinsic impacts [13, 14].

Gene products associated with treatment resistance or poor prognosis may be up or downregulated by these variables.

2.2.2 Tumor Microenvironment

Drug resistance discussions are expanding to include the tumor microenvironment as a key player in the development of relapse and incurability in many malignancies. Multiple components, such as stromal cells (SC), extracellular matrix (ECM), and soluble substances, compose the tumor microenvironment (cytokines and growth factors). Mediating drug resistance is communication between tumor cells and stromal cells at the extracellular matrix (ECM) interface [15]. As a source of additional signals for tumor cell proliferation, the tumor microenvironment, which contains GF and cytokines, plays a critical role in tumor development, progression, and survival. Some molecules may be included in the category of "environment-mediated drug resistance" (EM-DR) [15–17]. These molecules include vascular endothelial growth factor (VEGF), basic fibroblast growth factor (bFGF), stromal cell-derived factor-1 (SDF-1), interleukin-6 (IL-6), and nitric oxide (NO).

2.2.3 Cancer Stem Cells

Several types of malignancy, including those of the blood and solid organs, may be driven by populations of cancer stem cells. It has been revealed that cancer stem cells have specialized systems for evacuating chemotherapy chemicals, which may contribute to their resistance to treatment. Increased expression of ATP-binding cassette (ABC) drug transporters, such as P-glycoprotein encoding ABCB1 and mitoxantrone resistance-associated ABCG2. To prolong their lives, cancer stem cells are thought to share many characteristics with normal stem cells, including a low level of activity, resistance to drugs and toxins due to the expression of drug efflux transporters, an active DNA-repair capacity and resistance to cell death, and enhanced activity of repair enzymes in the vascular niche [18–20]. From this chapter, the readers understands about cancer cell biology, these cells may either remain in the patient's body and prevent cancer from returning, or they may invade other organs and spread the disease. Therefore, it is critical to locate and destroy these hidden aggregations of cancer cells, which are responsible for driving the evolution of treatment resistance.

2.2.4 Inactivation of the Anticancer Drugs

Several mechanisms contribute to the effectiveness and activity of anticancer medicines. Drugs may become active as a result of modifications to their chemical characteristics brought about by interactions with proteins in the body. That is why cancer cells develop resistance to therapy [21]. Nucleoside cytarabine (AraC), used in cancer treatment, is phosphorylated several times to yield cytarabine triphosphate (AraC-triphosphate). When activated through phosphorylation, AraC is a lethal protein that kills cells. For the first few days, cancer cells are barely affected [22]. Cancer cells can develop resistance to AraC treatment if the proteins and enzymes along this pathway (phosphorylation processes) are altered or down-regulated [23].

A different class of anti-cancer drugs targets the MAPEG proteins, which are dispersed throughout the cytosol, mitochondria, and microsomes. Some members of this enzyme family may be able to remove pharmaceuticals, ionizing substances, and electron compounds from the body. Drug resistance in cancer cells is facilitated both directly, through GST enzymes' detoxification of anti-cancer medications, and indirectly, via GST enzymes' inhibition of the MAPK pathway in the RAS–MAPK pathway. The potentially lethal side effects of chemotherapeutic medications can be reduced by elevating GST expression in cancer cells. Furthermore, this is associated with the resistance to apoptosis generated by diverse stimuli.

2.2.5 Multi-Drug Resistance

Multi-drug resistance (MDR) describes cancer cells' ability to survive in the presence of a wide range of anti-cancer drugs (MDR). It is possible that an MDR mechanism might be generated by increasing the drug's extracellular release. In turn, this reduces the cells' capacity to take medicines [24].

2.2.6 Increasing the Release of Drugs Outside the Cell

Nutrients and other chemicals are shuttled across the membrane via a variety of transporters that rely on ATP. This protein is divided into four different regions: two transmembrane domains (TMDs), two cytoplasmic domains (Cys-Ds), and two ATP-binding cassette (ABC) domains [24]. The ABC family consists of MRP1, P-glycoprotein (PGP), and breast cancer-resistant protein (BCRP/ABCG2) [25]. As an ATP-binding multifunctional membrane transporter, P-glycoprotein (P-gp) is most commonly known as a chloride efflux pump. However, P-gp also transports other medicines across the membrane. The chemotherapy medications doxorubicin, vinblastine, and taxol are examples of them. As a final step, the agent is released into the community. The medication is released from the transporter when the second hydrolysis returns it to its initial form (Figure 2.2) [26, 27].

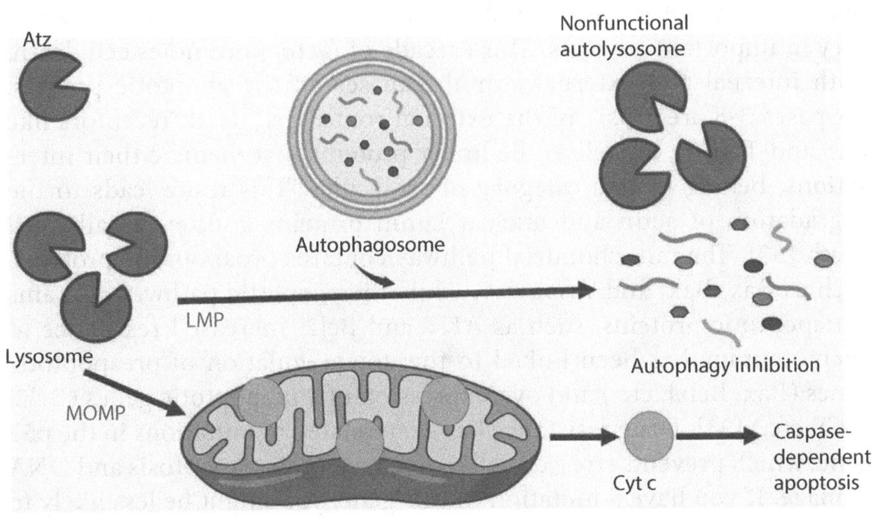

Figure 2.2 Schematic diagram of the mechanism of inhibition of the cell death.

2.2.7 Reducing the Absorption of the Drugs

Tumor cells may passively absorb nucleoside analogs (such as doxorubicin and vinblastine) (via mechanisms such as facilitating diffusion) [28]. The ABC transporter molecules allow all the noxious chemicals to enter the cells along the concentration gradient. However, active transport is required for cellular uptake when medicines are administered against a steep concentration gradient [29]. Solute carrier (SLC) proteins compose the vast majority of membrane transporters (transports minerals, vitamins, etc). Reduced drug absorption can be achieved in two ways: by reducing the number of transporters in the body or by decreasing the drug's binding propensity. Certain drugs enter cells with the help of transporters evolved for this purpose [30]. If these transporters are mutated, less medication is absorbed. A mutation in the human folate carrier (hRFC) gene is the most common cause of methotrexate resistance in patients with acute lymphoblastic leukemia (ALL). The affinity of the hRFC protein for drugs is decreased by a G-point mutation and glutamic acid substitution in the transmembrane region [31].

2.2.8 Inhibition of Cell Death (Apoptosis Pathway Blocking)

Necrosis, apoptosis, and autophagy are the three major mechanisms of cell death. All of these methods are biological in origin, yet they can vary in important respects. This cascade of factors promotes cell death. Both internal and external stimuli can set off the apoptotic process. Caspases 3-8 are a part of the external route. Cell death receptors like FAS and TNF-R, as well as the linker proteins that mediate their interactions, belong to this category of molecules. This route leads to the degradation of actin and nuclear lamin proteins and, eventually, cell death [32]. The mitochondrial pathway contains proapoptotic proteins, such as Bax, Bak, and caspase-9, while the apoptotic pathway contains antiapoptotic proteins, such as AKT and Bcl2. Increased resistance to chemotherapy has been linked to the downregulation of preapoptotic genes (Bax, Bclxl, etc.) and overexpression of antiapoptotic genes (Bcl2, AKT, etc.) [33]. Drug resistance has been related to mutations in the p53 gene, which prevents stressed cells from undergoing apoptosis and DNA damage. If you have a mutation in this gene, you might be less likely to experience apoptosis after experiencing DNA damage from chemotherapeutics [34].

2.3 Improving the Pharmacokinetics

Enzyme-catalyzed metabolism of chemotherapy drugs is possible. When comparing the inside-to-outside ratio of a substance, enzymes play a key role. Phase I activities, such as oxidation, reduction, and hydrolysis, and phase II reactions, such as consumption and conversion, are crucial for safeguarding healthy cells from hazardous chemicals. By decreasing enzyme activity and increasing the inactivation of prodrugs, cancer cells become less resistant to therapy (increased activity of some enzymes). Detoxification by cytochrome P450 is an excellent example of a phase I process that is regulated by cells [35]. The inactivation of docetaxel and the development of resistance to treatment in breast cancer have both been linked to increased cytochrome P450 activity [36]. However, it has been shown that reducing the activity of this enzyme improves therapeutic responsiveness. Its phase II reaction was transformed to glucuronic acid, sulphate, and glutathione, which decreased the medication's activity and abolished its electrophilic toxicity [37]. Anticancer medication resistance may be increased by upregulating glutathione synthesis and transferase-mediated glutathione detoxification.

2.4 Changing the Aim of the Chemotherapy Agents

Whether or if chemotherapeutic drugs affected their intended targets can be inferred from changes in expression levels, mutations, and other abnormalities. The development of drug resistance is inevitable if the agents' targets undergo such changes [38]. Examples include topoisomerase enzymes, which are used in DNA replication to unwind the twisted double helix [39]. Doxorubicin, an anthracycline fungal antibiotic, is the standard of care for treating solid tumors (such as breast cancer and lung tumors). Topoisomerase II activity may be inhibited. Topoisomerase II mutations in cancer cells reduce the drug's efficacy [40].

Drug resistance and changes in therapy targets are both driven by secondary mutations, which are common in chronic myelogenous leukemia (CML) and account for the disease's high imatinib resistance rate [41–44]. Translocation between the 3′ and 5′ ends of the ABL and BCR genes on chromosomes 9 and 22, respectively, causes Philadelphia chromosomes in CML.

There is currently no cure for BCR-ABL translocations since the particular sections of both genes involved depend on the location of the chromosomal breakpoint. The emergence of drug resistance results from a number of factors coming together. Point mutations and amino acid alterations in the BCR-kinase ABL domain disrupt the protein's native structure, making it difficult for medicines to bind [45–47].

There are about 70 distinct mutations in the kinase domain of BCR-ABL that have been discovered.

Changes to these 15 amino acids account for 80% to 90% of imatinib-resistant mutations. Y253, E255, T315, M351, F359, H396, and G250T account for 67% of all mutations. The vast majority of these cases are due to mutations in the A-Loop (A-Loop), C-Loop (C-Loop), P-Loop (P-Loop), or "Drug Contact site" (the binding site of imatinib).

The level of Imatinib resistance is based on the presence of mutations. The M351 mutation, for instance, is associated with a modest degree of imatinib resistance. Imatinib is not working at its current dose. Treatments of the first generation have not been effective against T315, V299L mutations (dasatinib). To treat Y253, E255 P-Loop mutations, doctors often use nilotinib, second-generation imatinib.

The structural alterations brought on by the point mutations that cause CML (Missense) may prohibit the protein from binding to the ATP-binding site of imatinib. Since the protein's activity as a tyrosine kinase is greatly increased and maintained [48–50]. Various disease and their inhibited pathway shown in Table 2.1.

Table 2.1 Inhibition of disease and drug-resistant processes and pathways.

Disease	The inability to be treated with prescribed medication interruption of mechanisms and pathways
CML	Bacterial sensitivity to imatinib
Myeloproliferative disorders	JAK2
AML	Adhesion and Wnt pathway b-catenin expression SHIP mutations affect GSK-3b activity and adhesion. Activation of PI3-kinase and Akt
ALL	PTEN mutation, loss, or inactivation results in increased Akt and PI3K expression.
Other human neoplasia	As part of the Jak and STAT cascades AKT and PKB signaling Raf/MEK and PI3K/PTEN/Akt pathways Jak and STAT

2.5 Improving the DNA Repair Process

The ability of cancer cells to repair their DNA has long been suspected as a resistance mechanism to chemotherapy. These drugs may cause direct or indirect damage to the DNA of cancer cells, suggesting the existence of DNA repair systems. Cisplatin, for example, has been shown to directly cause DNA damage, which in turn causes tumor cell death [51]. The NER and homologous recombination repair processes in cancer cells are to blame for their resistance to these drugs (RRM). The ability of these medications to impede cancer cells' natural DNA repair processes is important to their efficacy. To increase the effectiveness of chemotherapy against cancer cells, DNA repair pathways must be inhibited. Targeting mutations and epigenetic silencing in DNA repair systems in malignant cells may prove to be an effective treatment strategy [52]. Doxorubicin resistance may result from elevated DNA repair and alkyltransferase (alkylating agent) activity [53].

2.5.1 Augmentation of a Gene

In roughly 10% of malignancies, especially leukemias, an amplified gene represents a mechanism of treatment resistance. Numerous forms of cancer cells, including leukemia, undergo gene amplification, which increases the number of target genes and ultimately causes resistance to methotrexate [54]. Multiple copies of the drug-resistant dihydrofolate reductase gene are expressed by cancer cells (could target the enzyme of methotrexate). The number of oncogene copies in a cell may increase by a factor of several hundred during the amplification process. As a result, the body produces more of the associated oncoproteins [55]. Amplifications in cancer cells can be detected using a technique called homogeneously staining regions (HSR) or double chromosomes (double minute chromosomes [DMs]) [56].

2.5.2 Epigenetic Altering Caused Drug Resistance

Patients with cancer have developed resistance to chemotherapy due to epigenetic alterations. Examples of epigenetic alterations are DNA methylation and chromatin modifications [57]. When a methyltransferase attaches to the 5′ carbon of cytosine in CpG islands, DNA methylation takes place (upstream of the promoters). Methylation may take place at various additional sites across the genome as well [58]. Specific lysine residues at the ends of histones and non-histone proteins are acetylated by histone acetyltransferases (HATs) and deacetylases (HDACs), respectively. Alterations in chromatin structure and content may be facilitated by enzymes like these. Changes in lysine acetylation and deacetylation, respectively, regulate gene expression by either relaxing or tightening chromatin, respectively. 50 Methylation is commonly used to silence tumor suppressor genes while boosting the expression of oncogenes [59]. Demethylation of the multi-drug resistance gene (MDR1) causes a more drug-resistant phenotype in cancer cell lines by decreasing the accumulation of antitumor drugs within tumor cells. However, early myeloid cancer cells overexpress MDR1, while more advanced myeloid cancer cells downregulate it [60].

The epigenetic process may have an effect on their DNA repair mechanism. It is the job of mismatch repair proteins like HMLH1 and HMS1 and others to fix mistakes in DNA. The promoters of the following genes have been mutated or hypermethylated, making them cancer-causing. Mutations or hypermethylation of the hMLH1 gene, for instance, have been linked to the development of colorectal cancer [61]. 5-Aza-2′-deoxycytidine (decitabine) blocks DNA methylation but has minimal effect on tumor growth; instead, it makes tumors more vulnerable to chemotherapeutic agents like cisplatin and carboplatin.

By demethylating the hMLH1 promoter gene with DAC, the mismatch repair mechanism is reinstated, making colorectal cancer cells more sensitive to 5-FU [62].

Combinations of epigenetic and traditional chemotherapeutic medicines may be employed to attack tumors and cancer cells that have developed resistance [63].

2.6 MicroRNA in Cancer Drug Resistance

The miRNA family is comprised of two distinct RNA hairpin structures, with each containing around 22 nucleotides [64]. MicroRNAs are RNA molecules that influence gene expression but lack the coding sequence needed to produce a protein [65]. Many protein-coding genes are under their control, including those that cause cancer and those that are resistant to treatment. There are three pathways involved in miRNA-mediated gene silencing: Destabilizing the mRNA by shortening its poly(A) tail causes it to be cleaved into two segments, making protein translation by ribosomes less efficient [66].

Recent research in miRNA profiling has revealed the importance of these small molecules in determining whether a tumor would be sensitive or resistant to chemotherapy. To some extent, miRNA may be involved in each of the aforementioned drug-resistance processes [67]. Depending on the context, miRNAs can improve tumor responsiveness to chemotherapeutic treatments or prevent the development of resistance to cancer drugs. These compounds' potential as a biomarker for therapy efficacy and prognosis is intriguing.

2.7 Conclusion

Researchers have found that when antibiotics are used excessively, bacteria develop resistance to them. Due to the rapid cell division and mutation rate of these bacteria, resistant strains have developed through natural selection. Moreover, a high rate of proliferation in cancer cells is associated with genetic instability, which might in turn result in resistance to treatment. The cell biology of tumors can be changed, as has been shown in studies, to create cells that are smart and resistant to cellular stressors and agents. Several factors contribute to the complexity of the problem of cancer patients developing resistance to treatment. For cancers that have become resistant to multiple drugs, combination therapy is the best option. The researcher's investigated multiple mechanisms contributing to drug resistance, and concluded that combining epigenetic therapies with existing chemotherapeutic drugs in order to create a synergistic effect could be an effective new strategy for treating drug-resistant cancers. New research suggests that the RNA interference (RNAi) technique (especially siRNA) reduced and restricted drug resistance in the resistant tumoral cells, making the cancer cells more vulnerable to chemotherapeutic treatments. Therapeutic strategies that use miRNAs include miRNA replacement and miRNA masking. Specifically, this can be achieved by either reintroducing the tumor suppressor miRNA or blocking the target genes that contribute to cancer development or cancer drug resistance. In addition to conventional chemotherapy, RNA interference (RNAi)-based medicines like siRNA and miRNA may be effective against drug-resistant tumor cells.

References

1. MacConaill, L.E. and Garraway, L.A., Clinical implications of the cancer genome. *J. Clin. Oncol.*, 28, 35, 5219–28, 2010.

2. Goldenberg, M.M., Trastuzumab, a recombinant DNA-derived humanized monoclonal antibody, a novel agent for the treatment of metastatic breast cancer. *Clin. Ther.*, 21, 2, 309–18, 1999.
3. Longley, D.B. and Johnston, P.G., Molecular mechanisms of drug resistance. *J. Pathol.*, 205, 2, 275–92, 2005.
4. Goodman, L.S., Wintrobe, M.M., Dameshek, W., Goodman, M.J., Gilman, A., McLennan, M.T., Nitrogen mustard therapy: Use of methyl-bis (beta-chloroethyl) amine hydrochloride and tris (beta-chloroethyl) amine hydrochloride for hodgkin's disease, lymphosarcoma, leukemia and certain allied and miscellaneous disorders. *JAMA*, 132, 3, 126–32, 1946.
5. Barinaga, M., From bench top to bedside. *Science*, 278, 5340, 1036–9, 1997.
6. Nabholtz, J.M. and Slamon, D., New adjuvant strategies for breast cancer: Meeting the challenge of integrating chemotherapy and trastuzumab (herceptin). *Semin. Oncol.*, 28, 1 Suppl 3, 1–12, 2001.
7. Kreitman, R.J., Immunotoxins for targeted cancer therapy. *AAPS J.*, 8, 3, E532–51, 2006.
8. Benner, S.E., Wahl, G.M., Von Hoff, D.D., Double minute chromosomes and homogeneously staining regions in tumors taken directly from patients versus in human tumor cell lines. *Anticancer Drugs*, 2, 1, 11–25, 1991.
9. Arora, V.K., Schenkein, E., Murali, R., Subudhi, S.K., Wongvipat, J., Balbas, M.D. *et al.*, Glucocorticoid receptor confers resistance to antiandrogens by bypassing androgen receptor blockade. *Cell*, 155, 6, 1309–22, 2013.
10. Gupta, P.B., Fillmore, C.M., Jiang, G., Shapira, S.D., Tao, K., Kuperwasser, C. *et al.*, Stochastic state transitions give rise to phenotypic equilibrium in populations of cancer cells. *Cell*, 146, 4, 633–44, 2011.
11. Brown, G.D. *et al.*, Hidden killers: Human fungal infections. *Sci. Transl. Med.*, 4, 165rv13, 2012.
12. Burke, J.E. *et al.*, A non-Dicer RNase III and four other novel factors required for RNAi-mediated transposon suppression in the human pathogenic yeast *C. neoformans*. *bioRxiv*, 9, 7, 2235–2244, 2019.
13. Calo, S. *et al.*, A non-canonical RNA degradation pathway suppresses RNAi-dependent epimutations in the human fungal pathogen *Mucor circinelloides*. *PLoS Genet.*, 13, e1006686, 2017.
14. Calo, S. *et al.*, Two distinct RNA-dependent RNA polymerases are required for initiation and amplification of RNA silencing in the basal fungus *Mucor circinelloides*. *Mol. Microbiol.*, 83, 379–94, 2012.
15. Calo, S. *et al.*, Antifungal drug resistance evoked via RNAi-dependent epimutations. *Nature*, 513, 555–8, 2014.
16. Carninci, P. *et al.*, The transcriptional landscape of the mammalian genome. *Science*, 309, 1559–1563, 2005.
17. Cervantes, M. *et al.*, A single argonaute gene participates in exogenous and endogenous RNAi and controls cellular functions in the basal fungus *Mucor circinelloides*. *PLoS One*, 8, e69283, 2013.

18. Chang, Z. *et al.*, Broad antifungal resistance mediated by RNAi-dependent epimutation in the basal human fungal pathogen *Mucor circinelloides. PLoS Genet.*, 15, e1007957, 2019.
19. Chen, Z. *et al.*, Epigenetic regulation: A new frontier for biomedical engineers. *Annu. Rev. Biomed. Eng.*, 19, 195–219, 2017.
20. Clapier, C.R. and Cairns, B.R., The biology of chromatin remodeling complexes. *Annu. Rev. Biochem.*, 78, 273–304, 2009.
21. Clapier, C.R. *et al.*, Mechanisms of action and regulation of ATP-dependent chromatin-remodelling complexes. *Nat. Rev. Mol. Cell Biol.*, 18, 407–422, 2017.
22. Cortes, A. *et al.*, Epigenetic silencing of *Plasmodium falciparum* genes linked to erythrocyte invasion. *PLoS Pathog.*, 3, e107, 2007.
23. Cortes, A. *et al.*, A view on the role of epigenetics in the biology of malaria parasites. *PLoS Pathog.*, 8, e1002943, 2012.
24. Cowen, L.E. and Lindquist, S., Hsp90 potentiates the rapid evolution of new traits: Drug resistance in diverse fungi. *Science*, 309, 2185–9, 2005.
25. Cowen, L.E. *et al.*, Mechanisms of antifungal drug resistance. *Cold Spring Harb. Perspect. Med.*, 5, a019752, 2014.
26. de Haro, J.P. *et al.*, A single dicer gene is required for efficient gene silencing associated with two classes of small antisense RNAs in *Mucor circinelloides. Eukaryot. Cell*, 8, 1486–97, 2009.
27. Dimond, A. and Fraser, P., Long noncoding RNAs Xist in three dimensions. *Science*, 341, 720–1, 2013.
28. Dumesic, P.A. *et al.*, Stalled spliceosomes are a signal for RNAi-mediated genome defense. *Cell*, 152, 957–68, 2013.
29. Feretzaki, M. *et al.*, Gene network polymorphism illuminates loss and retention of novel RNAi silencing components in the *Cryptococcus* pathogenic species complex. *PLoS Genet.*, 12, e1005868, 2016.
30. Fisher, M.C. *et al.*, Worldwide emergence of resistance to antifungal drugs challenges human health and food security. *Science*, 360, 739–742, 2018.
31. Aas, T., Borresen, A.L., Geisler, S., Smith-Sorensen, B., Johnsen, H., Varhaug, J.E. *et al.*, Specific P53 mutations are associated with *de novo* resistance to doxorubicin in breast cancer patients. *Nat. Med.*, 2, 811–814, 1996.
32. Apperley, J.F., Part I: Mechanisms of resistance to imatinib in chronic myeloid leukaemia. *Lancet Oncol.*, 8, 1018–1029, 2007.
33. Arber, N., Doki, Y., Han, E.K., Sgambato, A., Zhou, P., Kim, N.H. *et al.*, Antisense to cyclin D1 inhibits the growth and tumorigenicity of human colon cancer cells. *Cancer Res.*, 57, 1569–1574, 1997.
34. Atwood, S.X., Chang, A.L., Oro, A.E., Hedgehog pathway inhibition and the race against tumor evolution. *J. Cell Biol.*, 199, 193–197, 2012.
35. Balak, M.N., Gong, Y., Riely, G.J., Somwar, R., Li, A.R., Zakowski, M.F. *et al.*, Novel D761Y and common secondary T790M mutations in epidermal growth factor receptor-mutant lung adenocarcinomas with acquired resistance to kinase inhibitors. *Clin. Cancer Res.*, 12, 6494–6501, 2006.

36. Bardenheuer, W., Lehmberg, K., Rattmann, I., Brueckner, A., Schneider, A., Sorg, U.R. *et al.*, Resistance to cytarabine and gemcitabine and *in vitro* selection of transduced cells after retroviral expression of cytidine deaminase in human hematopoietic progenitor cells. *Leukemia*, 19, 2281–2288, 2005.
37. Bean, J., Riely, G.J., Balak, M., Marks, J.L., Ladanyi, M., Miller, V.A. *et al.*, Acquired resistance to epidermal growth factor receptor kinase inhibitors associated with a novel T854A mutation in a patient with EGFR-mutant lung adenocarcinoma. *Clin. Cancer Res.*, 14, 7519–7525, 2008.
38. Bidard, F.C., Vincent-Salomon, A., Gomme, S., Nos, C., De Rycke, Y., Thiery, J.P. *et al.*, Disseminated tumor cells of breast cancer patients: A strong prognostic factor for distant and local relapse. *Clin. Cancer Res.*, 14, 3306–3311, 2008.
39. Blencke, S., Ullrich, A., Daub, H., Mutation of threonine 766 in the epidermal growth factor receptor reveals a hotspot for resistance formation against selective tyrosine kinase inhibitors. *J. Biol. Chem.*, 278, 15435–15440, 2003.
40. Borsellino, N., Belldegrun, A., Bonavida, B., Endogenous interleukin 6 is a resistance factor for cis-diamminedichloroplatinum and etoposide-mediated cytotoxicity of human prostate carcinoma cell lines. *Cancer Res.*, 55, 4633–4639, 1995.
41. Borsellino, N., Bonavida, B., Ciliberto, G., Toniatti, C., Travali, S., D'Alessandro, N., Blocking signaling through the Gp130 receptor chain by interleukin-6 and oncostatin M inhibits PC-3 cell growth and sensitizes the tumor cells to etoposide and cisplatin-mediated cytotoxicity. *Cancer*, 85, 134–144, 1999.
42. Borst, P., Evers, R., Kool, M., Wijnholds, J., A family of drug transporters: The multi-drug resistance-associated proteins. *J. Natl. Cancer Inst.*, 92, 1295–1302, 2000.
43. Braun, S., Kentenich, C., Janni, W., Hepp, F., De Waal, J., Willgeroth, F. *et al.*, Lack of effect of adjuvant chemotherapy on the elimination of single dormant tumor cells in bone marrow of high-risk breast cancer patients. *J. Clin. Oncol.*, 18, 80–86, 2000.
44. Breivik, J., The evolutionary origin of genetic instability in cancer development. *Semin. Cancer Biol.*, 15, 51–60, 2005.
45. Bryant, H.E., Schultz, N., Thomas, H.D., Parker, K.M., Flower, D., Lopez, E. *et al.*, Specific killing of BRCA2-deficient tumours with inhibitors of poly(ADP-ribose) polymerase. *Nature*, 434, 913–917, 2005.
46. Cai, J., Weiss, M.L., Rao, M.S., In search of "stemness". *Exp. Hematol.*, 32, 585–598, 2004.
47. Campbell, P.J., Stephens, P.J., Pleasance, E.D., O'Meara, S., Li, H., Santarius, T. *et al.*, Identification of somatically acquired rearrangements in cancer using genome-wide massively parallel paired-end sequencing. *Nat. Genet.*, 40, 722–729, 2008.

48. Castells, M., Thibault, B., Delord, J.P., Couderc, B., Implication of tumor microenvironment in chemoresistance: Tumor-associated stromal cells protect tumor cells from cell death. *Int. J. Mol. Sci.*, 13, 9545–9571, 2012.
49. Caulin, A.F. and Maley, C.C., Peto's Paradox: Evolution's prescription for cancer prevention. *Trends Ecol. Evol.*, 26, 175–182, 2011.
50. Chiarugi, A., A snapshot of chemoresistance to PARP inhibitors. *Trends Pharmacol. Sci.*, 33, 42–48, 2012.
51. Chin, L. and Gray, J.W., Translating insights from the cancer genome into clinical practice. *Nature*, 452, 553–563, 2008.
52. Costa, D.B., Halmos, B., Kumar, A., Schumer, S.T., Huberman, M.S., Boggon, T.J. *et al.*, BIM mediates EGFR tyrosine kinase inhibitor-induced apoptosis in lung cancers with oncogenic EGFR mutations. *PLoS Med.*, 4, e315, 2007.
53. Crespi, B. and Summers, K., Evolutionary biology of cancer. *Trends Ecol. Evol.*, 20, 545–552, 2005.
54. Croix, B.S., Rak, J.W., Kapitain, S., Sheehan, C., Graham, C.H., Kerbel, R.S., Reversal by hyaluronidase of adhesion-dependent multicellular drug resistance in mammary carcinoma cells. *J. Natl. Cancer Inst.*, 88, 1285–1296, 1996.
55. Damaraju, V.L., Damaraju, S., Young, J.D., Baldwin, S.A., Mackey, J., Sawyer, M.B. *et al.*, Nucleoside anticancer drugs: The role of nucleoside transporters in resistance to cancer chemotherapy. *Oncogene*, 22, 7524–7536, 2003.
56. Druker, B.J., Talpaz, M., Resta, D.J., Peng, B., Buchdunger, E., Ford, J.M. *et al.*, Efficacy and safety of a specific inhibitor of the BCR–ABL tyrosine kinase in chronic myeloid leukemia. *N. Engl. J. Med.*, 344, 1031–1037, 2001.
57. Engelhardt, B. and Kappos, L., Natalizumab: Targeting alpha4-integrins in multiple sclerosis. *Neurodegener. Dis.*, 5, 16–22, 2008.
58. Engelman, J.A., Zejnullahu, K., Mitsudomi, T., Song, Y., Hyland, C., Park, J.O. *et al.*, MET amplification leads to gefitinib resistance in lung cancer by activating ERBB3 signaling. *Science*, 316, 1039–1043, 2007.
59. Farmer, H., Mccabe, N., Lord, C.J., Tutt, A.N., Johnson, D.A., Richardson, T.B. *et al.*, Targeting the DNA repair defect in BRCA mutant cells as a therapeutic strategy. *Nature*, 434, 917–921, 2005.
60. Ferrantini, M., Capone, I., Belardelli, F., Interferon-alpha and cancer: Mechanisms of action and new perspectives of clinical use. *Biochimie*, 89, 884–893, 2007.
61. Frassanito, M.A., Cusmai, A., Iodice, G., Dammacco, F., Autocrine interleukin-6 production and highly malignant multiple myeloma: Relation with resistance to drug-induced apoptosis. *Blood*, 97, 483–489, 2001.
62. Frei, E. III, Karon, M., Levin, R.H., Freireich, E.J., Taylor, R.J., Hananian, J. *et al.*, The effectiveness of combinations of antileukemic agents in inducing and maintaining remission in children with acute leukemia. *Blood*, 26, 642–656, 1965.

63. Galmarini, C.M., Mackey, J.R., Dumontet, C., Nucleoside analogues: Mechanisms of drug resistance and reversal strategies. *Leukemia*, 15, 875–890, 2001.
64. Gatti, L. and Zunino, F., Overview of tumor cell chemoresistance mechanisms. *Methods Mol. Med.*, 111, 127–148, 2005.
65. Gioeli, D., *Targeted therapies mechanisms of resistance*, Humana Press, New York, 2011.
66. Giona, F., Testi, A.M., Annino, L., Amadori, S., Arcese, W., Camera, A. *et al.*, Treatment of primary refractory and relapsed acute lymphoblastic leukaemia in children and adults: The GIMEMA/AIEOP experience. Gruppo Italiano Malattie Ematologiche Maligne dell'Adulto. Associazione Italiana Ematologia ed Ocologia Pediatrica. *Br. J. Haematol.*, 86, 55–61, 1994.
67. Goldman, J.M. and Melo, J.V., Chronic myeloid leukemia - Advances in biology and new approaches to treatment. *N. Engl. J. Med.*, 349, 1451–1464, 2003.

3

Molecular Mechanism of Multi-Drug Resistant Cancer Cells

Rishabha Malviya*, Arun Kumar Singh and Deepika Yadav

Abstract

Acquiring resistance to chemotherapy is one of the biggest roadblocks to using it effectively in cancer treatment. Cancer is treated with a wide variety of anticancer methods, such as chemotherapy, radiation therapy, surgery, and targeted treatments. However, cancer cells reprogram themselves in a number of ways to escape the effects of these therapies, and ultimately the medication becomes inactive due to the development of multi-drug resistance (MDR). Cancer cells may develop the ability to live after being repeatedly exposed to anticancer therapies yet remain unaffected by the drugs themselves; this phenomenon is known as malignant drug resistance. The author summarized the current understanding of the molecular and cellular paradigms of MDR in cancer.

***Keywords*:** Multi-drug resistance, reactive oxygen, medication resistance, mechanism of drug resistance, glycoprotein

3.1 Introduction

From a societal and financial perspective, cancer is the second leading killer worldwide. There will likely be an uptick in cancer incidence and mortality rates in the coming years [1, 2]. Even though there have been significant improvements in cancer treatment over the years, there are still obstacles and unmet expectations. Chemotherapy and surgical procedures are two of the most common hospital cancer treatments, but cancer cells rapidly develop resistance to these procedures. Developing resistance to anticancer drugs is a significant matter. It is well known that chemotherapy has potential drawbacks, including systemic toxicity, immunological surveillance, and drug

**Corresponding author*: rishabhamalviya19@gmail.com

Rishabha Malviya, Arun Kumar Singh and Deepika Yadav. Multi-Drug Resistance in Cancer: Mechanism and Treatment Strategies, (47–76) © 2023 Scrivener Publishing LLC

resistance. The Food and Drug Administration has greenlit a broad variety of chemotherapy medications, the majority of which have a low molecular weight and hence need larger doses to exhibit their pharmacological effects. As a result, many anticancer medications attack chemicals that are present in both malignant and healthy cells [3–6]. Though chemotherapy initially proves successful against many types of cancer, many tumors develop resistance to it over time owing to both internal and environmental reasons. Examples include DNA damage repair mechanism changes, avoidance of programmed cell death, epithelial–mesenchymal transdifferentiation, and alterations to p53 expression, as well as cellular reprogramming, oncogenic stimulation, drug efflux due to overexpression of MDR genes and metabolic changes that promote drug inactivation and inhibition, and DNA damage repair mechanism changes [5]. Cancer cells may be able to avoid cell death in unforeseen ways, which may impede immune surveillance [6], while much research addressing the relationship between cancer and oxidative stress gives more evidence for the crucial role of ROS in cancer formation [7–10]. A major factor in the evolution of cancer treatment resistance is also the alteration of redox equilibrium. In addition to being crucial for cell viability, oxidative stress has been linked to treatment resistance in cancer patients.

Single-agent resistance occurs when the patient's cancer cells no longer respond to a single type of treatment, while multiagent resistance occurs when the cancer cells no longer respond to any type of anticancer drug (multi-drug resistance [MDR]).

Because they can thwart treatment goals, cancer patients who develop resistance to multiple medications have long been considered a "clinician's nightmare." Medication resistance is therefore a major challenge for any cancer treatment plan. The purpose of this research is to shed light on the various ways in which cancer cells have learned to evade treatment in order to stay alive [11, 12].

3.2 Types of Drug Resistance

Medication resistance is a complex problem with multiple causes, some innate and some learned. A patient's inherent resistance to a chemotherapeutic agent is referred to as "intrinsic resistance." 10 Multiple mechanisms, such as (a) innate genetic mutations in the tumor cells, (b) the emergence of a resistant population, such as cancer stem cells, in heterogeneous tumors, and (c) the initiation of intrinsic pathways that are responsible for detoxification under normal physiological conditions, have been proposed to explain how tumors can develop intrinsic resistance [13–15].

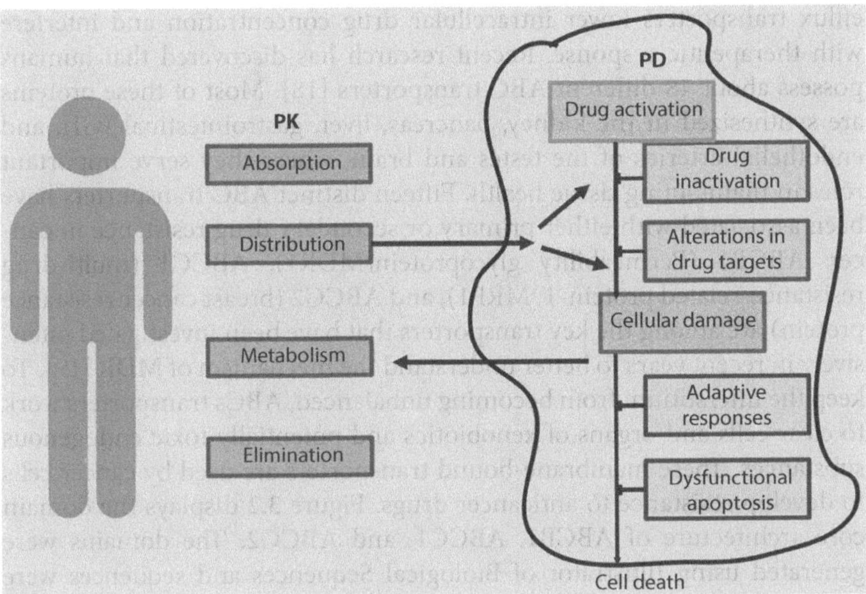

Figure 3.1 Molecular and cellular mechanisms leading to cancer medication resistance.

Despite this, acquired resistance may develop after cancer drugs have been used to treat the disease. Many cellular and molecular responses can lead to cancer cells becoming resistant to targeted drugs. These include (a) the activation of a second protooncogene following treatment, (b) changes in drug candidates, (c) drug metabolisms in the tumor, (d) efflux of drugs by membrane-spanning transporters (ATP binding cassettes, ABCs transporters), and (e) epigenomic alteration [16, 17].

Each of these drug-resistance pathways may contribute to multi-drug resistance in cancer, either independently or in combination.

This chapter provides a concise summary of the main cellular and molecular processes that contribute to cancer's resistance to treatment (Figure 3.1).

3.3 Mechanisms of Drug Resistance

3.3.1 Drug Efflux via ABC Transporters

Cancer drug resistance is tightly regulated by the overexpression of ABC transporter proteins. These transporters efflux substrates with a wide range of structural and functional characteristics through the cell membrane by hydrolyzing ATP [17]. Chemotherapy is less effective because drug efflux transporters lower intracellular drug concentration and interfere with therapeutic response. Recent research has discovered that humans possess about 48 different ABC transporters [18]. Most of these proteins are synthesized in the kidney, pancreas, liver, gastrointestinal (GI), and endothelial arteries of the testes and brain, where they serve important roles in maintaining tissue health. Fifteen distinct ABC transporters have been associated with either primary or secondary drug resistance in cancer. ABCB1 (Permeability glycoprotein/MDR1), ABCC1 (multi-drug resistance-related protein-1, MRP1), and ABCG2 (breast cancer resistance protein) are among the key transporters that have been investigated intensively in recent years to better understand the mechanism of MDR [19]. To keep the interstitium from becoming unbalanced, ABCs transporters work to clear cells and organs of xenobiotics and potentially toxic endogenous substances. These membrane-bound transporters are used by cancer cells to develop resistance to anticancer drugs. Figure 3.2 displays the domain core architecture of ABCB1, ABCC1, and ABCG2. The domains were generated using Illustrator of Biological Sequences and sequences were retrieved from Uniprot Database17 (IBS) [20].

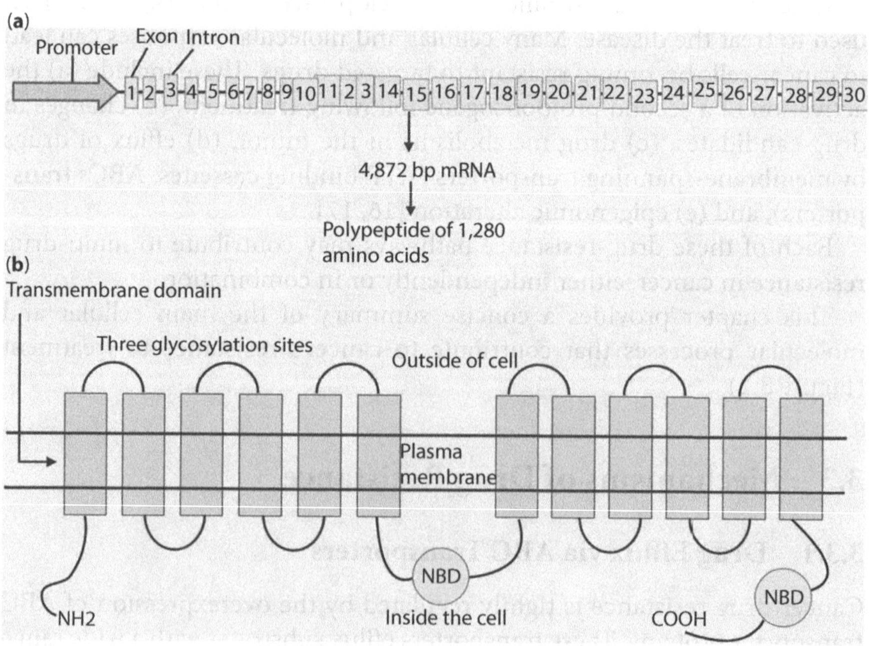

Figure 3.2 Schematic representation of the structural organization of ABCB1, ABCC1, and ABCG2. (a) Linear structure of mRNA stand showing entron and exon with promotor, (b) Schematic diagram of a typical ABC transporter.

This class of ABC transporters relies heavily on ATP for the regulation of their activities. Cancer cells that have developed resistance to chemotherapy produce more ATP than their nonresistant counterparts. The cancer cells become more susceptible to treatment when their ATP levels drop. Conversely, cells with elevated ATP levels change from being sensitive to drugs to being resistant to them. Drug efflux is increased because extracellular ATP increases the expression of ABC transporters [21]. TME is bolstered by rising levels of ATP outside of cells [5]. Cancer cells use a process called macropinocytosis to absorb the extra ATP [22]. Thus, the dramatic increase in intracellular ATP concentration causes the emergence of multi-drug resistance. The author discussed about the primary transporters that facilitate the elimination of chemotherapeutic drugs from the body, or efflux [23–28].

3.3.2 Permeability Glycoprotein/MDR-1

P-glycoprotein (P-gp) is a prototypical human ABC transporter since it was the first plasma membrane glycoprotein identified (encoded by the ABCB1 [adenosine Triphosphate binding cassette, subfamily B, member 1] gene). The gene for ABCB1 is found on human chromosome 7 and codes for a protein of around 170 kDa and 1280 amino acids [29–32]. Protein structure includes both a transmembrane domain (TMD) and a nucleotide-binding domain (NBD). In the cytosol, each P-gp subunit has a nucleotide-binding domain and six membrane-spanning helices in common [33]. This protein has a sizable, adaptable drug-binding pocket in its membrane-bound region. The pocket contains multiple putative binding subsites for the drug [34]. When ATP binds to the NBDs and is hydrolyzed, conformational changes in the TMDs switch the transporter from an intracellular to an extracellular state, allowing for unidirectional transport [35–40]. P-gp has to have some kind of interaction with the lipid-soluble proteins that it is trying to pump into the extracellular aqueous phase or translocate to the outer membrane leaflet because both of these processes need the proteins in question. P-gp defends against xenobiotics and harmful compounds and is expressed at a baseline level in many normal organs. These organs include the liver, colon, kidney, testes, placenta, and blood–brain barrier [41, 42]. The most-requested transporter proteins are P-gp transporters, which play a crucial role in drug-developing resistance in cancer cells. Many drug-resistant cancer cells show metabolic alterations, the most common of which is an increase in P-gp expression. Multi-drug-resistant cells have P-gp at their core because it inhibits the accumulation of chemotherapeutic drugs inside the cells [43, 44]. The P-gp is essential for intestinal transport and efflux, so it plays a role in modifying the bioavailability and therapeutic effects of medicines taken orally. Recent research suggests that P-gp overexpression in malignant neoplasms may play a role in the development of MDR [45]. Due to the substrate selectivity of P-broad gp, P-gp overexpressed cells may develop resistance to a wide range of potentially curative medications, a process known as multi-drug resistance (MDR) in cancer cells. Growing publications on P-gp have proven its influence on roughly 300 compounds, including the newly added "kinase inhibitors," which were originally assumed to be responsible for the uptake inhibition of common genotoxic anticancer medications like vinblastine, paclitaxel, and doxorubicin [46]. Cancer cells, in order to protect themselves from cytotoxic substances, generate P-gp. In addition, cancer cells that have been repeatedly exposed to chemotherapeutic drugs produce P-gp, which is then used to efflux the drug and decrease its levels within the cell [47, 48]. P-gp expression is also fostered by the disruption in cell-to-cell communication which is a characteristic of cancer. Cancer cells are able to upregulate P-gp expression for the goal of subverting drug function with considerable assistance from tumor hypoxia, the Warburg effect, and acidosis in the tumor microenvironment (TME) [49]. The simultaneous activation of multiple genes in response to oncogenic activation, epigenetic alterations, and abnormal cell death signaling allows cancer cells to acquire resistance to drugs. The rapid progression of multi-drug resistance in cancer has been related to the expression of P-gp in MDR cells, which is responsible for the efflux of anticancer medicines from the nucleus and mitochondria into the cytosol [50].

3.3.3 Multi-Drug Resistance Protein

The Multi-drug Resistance Protein (MRPs/ABCC1) protein, which has a molecular weight of 190 kDa, is made up of three hydrophobic transmembrane domains (TMD) with seventeen membrane-spanning helices, two N-terminal domains (NBD), and an extra N-terminal domain [51–55]. The ABC transporter 30 P-gp is only one of 13. Tumor cells have been shown to generate members of the multi-drug resistance-associated protein (MRP) family 1-9, and their expression levels have been found to correlate with resistance to anticancer treatments [56]. MRP consists of 3 TMD and 2 NBD. MDR cells lacking P-gp expressed MRP1/ABCC1. Like P-gp, MRP1 utilizes adenosine triphosphate (ATP) to speed up the removal of potentially hazardous substances.33 Proximal tubules in the kidney are where MRP is most abundant and where it plays a critical role in the excretion process [57]. MRP1 is continuously expressed in the placenta, kidneys, and testes, and is also detectable in the blood. However, MRP1 expression was significantly upregulated in several malignancies, including those of the lung, pancreas, prostate, brain, and breast [58]. MRP1 is essential for the elimination of several anticancer medicines, including anthracyclines, vinca alkaloids, methotrexate, camptothecins, and epipodophyllotoxins, as well as glucuronide, sulfate, and glutathione conjugates. Furthermore, low-oxygen conditions encourage MRP1 expression. In colon cancer cells, the literature showed a correlation between HIF-1 and MRP1 expression. However, cancer cells are more likely to produce MRP1 because of MDR activation by a collection of proteins that are exclusive to cancer cells [59].

3.3.4 Breast Cancer Resistance Protein

Breast cancer resistance protein (BCRP/ABCG2) is a transporter protein that, under normal physiological conditions, learns to eliminate potentially harmful chemicals from the extracellular spaces. It has a molecular weight of around 72 kDa and is made up of a single TMD and a single NBD. This protein is primarily expressed in stem cells and the apical membranes of the epithelium, where it plays a role in the degradation of unwanted drugs [60]. It is also found on the luminal surface of endothelial cells lining the cerebral capillaries, in addition to the usual suspects like the breast, adrenal gland, placenta, prostate, and kidney. Mitoxantrone resistance protein (ABCG2) is another name for ABCG2 due to its function in mitoxantrone efflux in carcinoma cells (MXR) [61–65]. One way in which cancer cells avoid death by cytotoxic drugs is through the upregulation of BCRP expression [66]. Cancer drugs, such as tyrosine kinase inhibitors and standard genotoxic agents, are rendered ineffective by BCRP chemoresistance. There is growing evidence that BCRP is present in other malignancies, such as leukemia and lung cancer, in addition to breast cancer, which is where it was initially identified [67]. It may be used as a marker for cancer stem cells in certain cancers. Many chemotherapeutic drugs, such as epipodophyllotoxin, mitoxantrone, camptothecins, bisantrene, anthracyclines, flavopiridol, and the tyrosine kinase inhibitors gefitinib and imatinib, may be transported effectively by ABCG2 [68–72]. The overexpression of these drug efflux transporters is a major driving force behind the development of multi-drug resistance in cancerous tumors. The roles of ABCB1, ABCC1, and ABCG2 and their associated genes in cancer were discussed. Researchers looked up information about the proteins of interest and the proteins with which they interact in the STRING database version [73, 74] and analyzed the genes of these interacting partner proteins using the Comparative Toxicogenomics Database (CTD)43 and

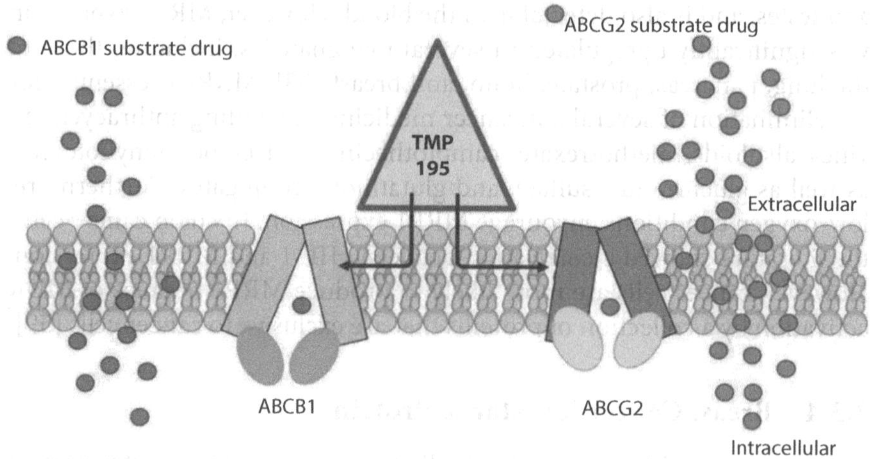

Figure 3.3 Cancer-related genes ABCB1, ABCC1, and ABCG2 interact with one another.

discovered that they all participate in cancer pathogenesis (details are not included in this review and can be found in CTD by gene name). Figure 3.2 displays the molecular action and network views, respectively, illustrating the inhibition and activation of interaction partners by the protein of interest. Interaction of Cancer related gene is shown in Figure 3.3.

3.4 Reduction in Drug Activity and Cellular Absorption

The drug's systemic distribution and absorption regulate its cellular activity and reaction. The vast array of drug-metabolizing enzymes in the human body facilitates the biochemical transformation of drugs once they enter the body [75]. Several anticancer drugs rely on metabolic activation for their antitumor mechanism of action. However, if there is a mutation or change in the enzymes responsible for drug metabolism, the drug will become inactive [76]. Drugs are activated and inactivated in cancer cells through the cytochrome P450 (CYP) system, the glutathione-S-transferase (GST) superfamily, and the uridine diphospho-glucuronosyltransferase (UGT) superfamily. It is the cytochrome P450 (CYP) enzyme that aids in the metabolism of bile acids, fatty acids, human steroid hormones, and lipid-soluble vitamins. Of the more than 57 CYPs discovered in human microsomes, 15 have been linked to the metabolism of various drugs [77]. The effectiveness with which these proteins metabolize and release the medication may be affected by variations in CYP. This would lead to a gradual decrease in the concentration of the medicine within tumors, thereby rendering the therapy ineffective [78]. The breast cancer prevention and treatment drug tamoxifen, for instance, loses its efficacy when the CYP2D6 gene is mutated or altered. Reduced drug absorption is another potential method by which cancer cells acquire resistance to therapy. Drugs are taken up by cells via endocytosis or receptor-mediated endocytosis; if either of these processes breaks down, drug resistance can develop. Caveolin-1 (CAV1) expression is related to tumor progression and the capacity to metastasize. Important in changing the relationship between tumor and host, it promotes metastasis, tumor development, treatment resistance, and cell survival [79].

In addition, the activation of detoxification mechanisms designed to protect against environmental contaminants may reduce the efficacy of anticancer drugs. Cancer cells that fail to properly detoxify their environment are the source of both poor treatment responses and subsequent resistance. Glutathione S-transferase may be responsible for much of the inability of cancer cells to rid themselves of drugs [80]. Glutathione S-transferase is essential for several cellular activities, such as cell division, cell fate determination, and cell death. An elevated glutathione (GSH) level is linked to drug resistance via multiple mechanisms. Previous studies suggest it may prevent cisplatin48 from working by interacting with reactive oxygen species (ROS), binding to medicines, preventing DNA/protein damage, or taking part in the DNA repair pathway. Doxorubicin plus 5-fluorouracil combination [81]. Medications may promote tumor growth by disrupting the normal balance of kinases due to an increase in GST. The promoter regions encoding for GCL and GST expression include binding sites for transcriptional regulators like AP-1, AP-2, NF-kB, and Nrf-2. In response to oxidative stress, the Nrf-2 transcription factor becomes dissociated from its negative regulator Keap [82–85]. It translocates to different parts of the cell and then forms a heterodimer with Maf proteins, binding to the antioxidant response element (ARE) sequences (ARE). As a result of this binding, detoxifying and cytoprotective genes such as glutathione S-reductase (GSR), glutathione co-transferase (GST), glutathione S-transferase (GCLM), glutathione S-transferase (GCLC), glutathione S-transferase (GST), ferritin, myeloperoxidase (MRP), heme oxygen (NQO1). Multiple types of human cancer carry mutations in Nrf-2 and keap1, and these mutations promote treatment resistance by permanently activating Nrf-2 and leading to increased production of cytoprotective (prosurvival) genes [86]. Substrates like steroids, xenobiotics, bile acids, cytotoxics, and xenobiotics are converted into inactive hydrophilic glucuronides by the ubiquitin-conjugating enzyme (UGT) superfamily, which catalyzes glucuronidation. First-line metabolic defence against harmful substrates is encoded by the UGT1 and UGT2 genes and is essential for the survival of many human tissues. Malignant cells were found to have reduced levels of UGT1A1 transcription and microsomal activity. Irinotecan, an inhibitor of topoisomerase I, is ineffective without the presence of UDP-glucuronosyltransferase 1A1 (UGT1A1). This enzyme is negatively regulated by DNA methylation [87]. However, irinotecan resistance is promoted by epigenetic alterations that increase UGT1A1 expression (by inactivating the medication). Overall, more study is needed to pinpoint the inactivation mechanism that ultimately causes cancer cells to become resistant to treatment.

Numerous studies have connected therapy failure to a tumor's poor capacity to absorb and distribute medicines. Only if the prescribed dose is taken by the patient will the treatment be considered successful. Cancer cells and the tumor microenvironment (TME) employ a variety of strategies to prevent drug uptake. Studies have shown that low oxygen tension is optimal for cancer stem cells, creating a perfusion barrier that prevents the drug from reaching the diseased tissue. Clonal growth of cancer tissue is also a barrier to the development of adequate vasculature around sites where new tumors have formed. Because of this, less of the drug will reach the tumor. Drug delivery is severely hampered by the presence of an extracellular matrix (ECM), which serves as a physical barrier to drug penetration.

3.5 Instability in the Genome and Medication Resistance

3.5.1 Mutation and Medication Target Alteration

The involvement of DNA mutations in both the initiation and development of cancer is well established. Cancer can originate from a number of different cellular processes, including DNA mutations, chromosomal abnormalities, telomere damage, and the DNA repair system [86]. Recent research has highlighted the role of chromosomal instability in promoting neoplastic cell transformation, tumor heterogeneity, and acquired drug resistance, all of which have bearing on the efficacy of cancer treatment and the likelihood of patient survival. Mutations can occur at any level of biological organization, from the single nucleotide to the chromosome, and are frequently found in both solid tumors and hematological malignancies. However, it is conceivable that mutations or aberrant expression of therapeutic targets caused by genomic instability in cancer cells are the major drivers of acquired resistance to conventional treatments (genes or proteins). Anticancer medications lose some of their effectiveness when their cellular targets are altered, and this may also increase drug resistance [87–90]. There is mounting evidence that alterations in the oestrogen receptor of tumor cells contribute to tamoxifen resistance in breast cancer patients. 59 Different types of gene alterations acquired by cancer cells may lessen their sensitivity to chemotherapy. Clinical studies involving persons with chronic myelogenous leukemia have indicated that between 20% and 30% of those treated with the tyrosine kinase inhibitor (TKI) imatinib eventually develop resistance and recurrence. This is because the fusion tyrosine kinase protein has a point mutation in isoleucine (T315I). Mutations in the tumor suppressor gene p53 cause impaired function and an abnormal proapoptotic balance, exacerbating the problem of medication resistance. Two studies have shown that cisplatin resistance in non-small cell lung cancer (NSCLC) cells are caused by an increase in the expression of the transcription factor Nrf-2, which is activated in response to p53 mutations. Mutant p53's capacity to remain nuclear in response to drug treatment was a contributing factor in cancer cells' resistance to gemcitabine [91].

3.5.2 Restoration of DNA Integrity

Oncology practitioners have used drugs that cause DNA damage to induce cell death or mitotic catastrophe as a means of treating cancer [92]. Inducing DNA damage is how these medications operate, but the repair mechanism for this damage also leads to the development of resistance. DNA lesions, DSBs, and SSBs, as well as double-strand breaks, are all repaired by the DNA Damage Response (DDR) pathways working in tandem (DSBs). Nucleotide excision repair (NER), base excision repair (BER), nonhomologous end joining (NHEJ), mismatch repair (MMR), translesion synthesis (TLS), the Fanconi anemia (FA) route, and homologous recombination (HR) are all examples of such mechanisms (DSB) [93]. Mutant copies of these genes are often found in cancer cells, where they provide enhanced DNA repair ability and resistance to apoptosis. Chemotherapeutic medicines, such as 5-fluorouracil (5-FU) and cisplatin, may damage DNA in cancer cells. However, cancer cells develop resistance to therapy over time as a result of the overexpression of genes in the DNA repair pathway [94]. Previous studies have linked cisplatin resistance in cancer to a lack of p53 and DNA mismatch repair. Clinical studies showed that 5-fluorouracil (Fu)-resistant human colorectal cells had higher expression of DNA repair genes like RAD23B, FANCG, and FEN1. The inability of cancer cells to enter the cell cycle and the prevention of programmed cell death as a result of abnormal DNA damage repair systems are major contributors to the development of cancer drug resistance.

3.5.3 Resistant Genes and Epigenetic Modifications

Epigenetic regulation of genes is critical for pinpointing a disease's origin and identifying a cell's fate. The emergence of tumor-initiating cells and/or resistance to therapeutic interventions may be aided by nongenetic diversity. The defective gene expression brought on by epigenetic alterations is retained through cell division, helping to pave the way for the emergence of nongenetic heterogeneity and treatment resistance [95]. Changes in chromatin packaging, caused by epigenetic modifications, regulate the amount of DNA that can be accessed by transcription factors based on their specific DNA sequence of interest, thereby affecting gene transcription. Epigenetic modifications, such as DNA methylation, chromatin remodeling, histone modification, and abnormalities in noncoding RNA, have a role in cancer development. It has been shown that aberrant methylation of CpG islands in or around the promoter region of genes is associated with gene inactivation during tumor formation [71, 72]. After a gene's DNA is methylated 72 times, histone methyltransferases and histone deacetylases (HDACs) are recruited to the site. This results in histone modification, chromatin condensation, and transcriptional silence of the linked genes. The frequency of such epimutations is much higher than that of genetic mutations. Metastasis was found to be accompanied by the appearance of at least 61 rare mutations, 15 of which were determined to be driver genes and the remaining genes to be mutated passengers [96]. Accordingly, these alterations have an outsized impact on the selection of subpopulations that are linked to tumor growth and the emergence of resistance to chemotherapeutic drugs. The MDR1 promoter has been shown to be demethylated in many tumor cells, and this seems to be linked to the emergence of MDR. When this promoter is methylated, drug accumulation is decreased, transcription of MDR1 is controlled, and drug resistance is increased in cancer cells. Tumor cells' ability to survive and develop resistance to methylating chemotherapeutic agents is bolstered by epigenetic alterations that reactivate the DNA repair enzyme MGMT. Multiple studies have linked the methylation and epigenetic silencing of tumor suppressor genes like BRCA1 and E-cadherin as well as proapoptotic genes like APAF1 and hMLH1 to cancer cell resistance [97]. Furthermore, the exosome's significance in epigenetic alterations was supported by the present synthesis report. Exosomes have been linked to cancer, cell proliferation, and metastasis by some studies.

Histone modification, DNA methylation, and RNA posttranscriptional regulation are only some of the cellular processes that may be influenced by the transport of proteins and nucleic acids through extracellular vesicles [98]. Exosomes are released by fibroblasts and immunocytes in the TME, and they transport a vast variety of payloads and microRNAs (miRNAs). Drug resistance mechanisms are partially controlled by exosomal microRNAs [99]. Among them include drug efflux, metabolic modifications, target mutation, DNA damage repair, metabolic abnormalities, cancer stem cells, and epigenetic alterations. As a result, exosomal miRNAs are critical in the emergence of resistance to therapeutic interventions [100].

3.5.4 Drug Resistance and Programmed Cell Death

Cancer cells avoid their normal scheduled death to maintain an unmatched ability for multiplying. Cancer is characterized by abnormal apoptosis regulation. Mutations in apoptotic and antiapoptotic genes, as well as shifts in gene expression, may contribute to the emergence of drug resistance, according to recent studies [101]. It has been shown that antiapoptotic genes and proteins, including the Bcl-2 family, decoy receptors (such as TRAIL-R3/DcR1 and TRAIL-R4/DcR2), cFLIP, and inhibitors of apoptosis proteins (IAPs), have a role in chemotherapy resistance [102]. Multiple studies have linked increased expression of BCL2, BCL-XL, and MCL-1 with chemotherapy-induced drug resistance in cancer. A rise in the expression of death receptors such as TRAIL-R1, TRAIL-R2, and FAS has also been associated with resistance to chemotherapy [103]. There is a very intricate signaling system responsible for controlling when and how cells undergo programmed death. Cellular responses and cell fates in response to death or survival signals are mediated by multiple transcription factors, including nuclear factor kappa B (NF-kB), hypoxia-inducible factor 1 (HIF-1), c-myc, activating transcription factor 1 (AP-1) and signal transducer and activator of transcription 3 (STAT-3). Apoptosis, autophagy, and necroptosis are just some of the cell death mechanisms that chemotherapeutic drugs can trigger. Necrotic cell death, on the other hand, may trigger inflammation and survival signaling via nuclear translocation of NF-kB and the production of proinflammatory cytokines, while apoptosis lowers inflammation but is normally avoided by immune cells [104]. The TME and cellular viability are both improved by this treatment. When exposed to a drug, sensitive cells take measures, such as activating nuclear factor (NF)-kB, to protect themselves from the drug's harmful effects. When NF-kB is activated, it moves into the nucleus, where it activates the transcription factors that contribute to chemoresistance in cancer cells. There is a close relationship between the molecular principles of cell signaling and the pharmacological response. Cancer cells are killed by chemotherapy drugs because of their cytotoxic effects, which include boosting ROS production, changing mitochondrial membrane permeability, damaging DNA, turning on tumor suppressor genes and proteins, and modifying immune cells [105]. Cancer cells are able to adapt and proliferate due to several alterations at the molecular level. For instance, when the p53 gene is mutated, chemotherapy agents that normally induce p53-mediated apoptosis in cancer cells may have a reduced effect [106]. Higher levels of the antiapoptotic protein survivin are produced by cancer cells with resistance, possibly as a result of the downregulation of tumor suppressor genes. Cancer cells that overexpress survivin are more able to avoid cell death and are more resistant to chemotherapy. Since DNA damage is how cisplatin works, cancer cells with a DNA repair mechanism may develop resistance to the drug. Wip1 is a protein that was found in resistant cells and works to inhibit the ATM DNA damage response pathway. Next, Wip1 was knocked down to sensitize the cisplatin-resistant oral squamous cell carcinoma (SCC) cells. By interfering with apoptotic signals, P-gp expression provides "two-way" protection for cancer cells. Expression levels of p-gp are inversely proportional to those of TNF-related apoptosis-inducing ligands (TRAIL) [107]. P-gp expression in cancer cells has been shown to suppress apoptosis in transformed cells, according to recent research.

Additionally, environmental stresses can set off a process called autophagy, which is a form of programmed cell death [108]. To maintain homeostasis, cells engage in a process called autophagy, which is a lysosomal-mediated degradation system that eliminates defective organelles and cellular components [109]. Autophagy inhibits tumor development under normal physiological settings, but it has been linked to cell proliferation in cancer when it is abnormal. Autophagy's molecular process has shed light on how cells maintain constant energy levels in the face of nutritional shortage. To some extent, increased autophagic flow can promote cell survival by activating death signals. For survival, cancer cells require a constant supply of energy, which they obtain from the tissues of their patients. Nutritional depletion or the stress situation brought on by treatment for cancer can cause autophagic cell death, which can lead to a patient developing resistance to cytotoxic drugs. But the role of autophagy in treating cancer is still being discussed. A recently reported finding suggests that the autophagic response can shield cancer cells from the toxicity of chemotherapy. It is well established that autophagy promotes MDR in cancer cells [109, 110]. Blocking autophagy is a supporting mechanism that restores sensitivity to chemotherapeutic agents in previously chemoresistant cells. Increased resistance to chemotherapy, radiation, and even targeted treatments has been associated with elevated autophagy. Signaling pathways play a significant part in the regulation of autophagy-mediated MDR, with the precise function dependent on the intervention, the surrounding environment, and the kind of cancer being treated [111–115]. To provide just one example, the PI3K/Akt/mTOR pathway activates the HSP90AA1 gene in osteosarcoma cells, which promotes resistance to doxorubicin, methotrexate, and cisplatin. One of p62's various functions is in facilitating autophagy-mediated resistance to drugs [116]. Triple-resistant HEp-2 cells were shown to have increased levels of autophagy and decreased levels of p62, an antioxidant protein, in a separate investigation. Autophagy induced by oxidative stress was blocked in cells with low p62 levels, high Nrf-2 levels, and high autophagic flux [117]. Some studies have shown that Sorafenib resistance is associated with overexpression of p62 in human hepatocarcinoma (HCC) cells. This finding may reflect how the function of p62 shifts with different cancer types and treatment options. Some cancer cells acquire resistance through a process called IL-6–mediated autophagy. Interleukin-6 (IL-6) activation and the following autophagic response in resistant cells are triggered by transglutaminase 2 (TG2)-mediated constitutive activation of nuclear factor-kappa B. According to the available evidence, IL-6–mediated autophagy is activated via a positive loop mechanism that results in the release of ATG5, an autophagic protein essential for autophagosome formation [98]. Autophagy may play a major role in determining how well cancer cells respond to radiation or ionization therapy. Furthermore, autophagy has been identified as a mediator of radiation treatment resistance in breast cancer. A tumor suppressor protein called liver kinase B1 (LKB1) was found in another study to be responsible for cancer cell radiation resistance. By activating AMP-activated protein kinase (AMPK), LKB1 suppressed apoptosis in resistant cells while promoting autophagy [118–120]. Restricting autophagy while simultaneously activating apoptosis after cancer cells have been exposed to various treatments may be beneficial in preventing them from changing from a sensitive to a resistant phenotype.

Uncontrolled cell death is called necrosis. Visually resembling necrosis and mechanically resembling apoptosis, necroptosis has been considered a form of caspase-independent, programmed cell death [121]. Research suggests that necrotic cells produce HMGB1, a crucial necrotic component that activates the inflammatory signaling cascade and aids in the formation of TME [122]. The nuclear protein HMGB1 is a vital component of cellular homeostasis and is covalently bound to chromatin. Although it can be found in both the nucleus and cytoplasm, its primary location is in the nucleus. As a chemical signal, HMGB1 encourages and exacerbates the inflammatory response that assists in the development and spread of cancer. Necrosis is a response to stress that results in the release of a crucial regulator of cell death and survival signaling from stressed cells [123]. It has been shown that chemo-exposed cancer cells secrete HMGB1, which has been shown in other studies to promote cell survival and drug resistance [124]. Unfortunately, necrosis causes the release of danger-associated molecular pattern molecules (DAMPs), which activate inflammasome components and lead to the secretion of proinflammatory cytokines like interleukin (IL)-1, IL-18, and tumor necrosis factor (TNF), all of which contribute to an inflammatory TME that aids resistance to anticancer therapy [125]. Since the inception of cancer research, scientists have known that chronic inflammatory responses play a pivotal role in the progression of many different cancer types. Release of the danger signaling protein HMGB1 may activate dendritic cells (DCs) and other immune cells via Toll-like receptor (TLR), rash-associated gene (RAGE), and nuclear factor (NF)-kappa B (NF-kappa B) signaling. Thus, our findings support the hypothesis that faulty programmed cell death signaling contributes to the development of drug resistance in cancer.

3.6 RNA Interference Therapy

Highly targeted therapeutic approaches for cancer treatment have lately been the focus of research into gene-silencing technologies based on small interfering RNA (siRNA) constructs, short hairpin RNAs, or antisense oligodeoxynucleotides at the mRNA level [126–130]. Small interfering RNAs (siRNAs) are used to inhibit the activity of drug-resistant genes like P-gp/MDR1, MRP1, Bcl2, BCRP, and others involved in multidrug resistance. However, these architectures are not at their therapeutic peak. Therefore, siRNA encapsulation into nanoparticles is very effective because it prevents the rapid destruction of siRNA molecules in serum, limits exposure to normal cells, increases the selectivity of cellular targets, and enhances cellular uptake. Unaltered siRNA is eliminated from circulation via degradation and renal excretion within minutes. When siRNAs are encapsulated in nanoparticles, however, only 30% of the siRNA is cleared from the bloodstream within 30 minutes. Through the use of a ligand-functionalized liposomal formulation, 20% of the administered siRNA was detected in the bloodstream 24 hours after treatment [131]. Liposomes, dendrimers, micelles, and silica are just a few examples of nanoparticle compositions utilized to carry both siRNA and chemotherapeutic medicines. Expression of the MDR1 gene was significantly silenced, topoisomerase II was inhibited, doxorubicin was intercalated, and resistant tumors shrank due to transcriptional inhibition and tumor regression when C-Myc siRNA was combined with doxorubicin-loaded cationic and anionic liposome poly cation-DNA nanoparticles. Dendrimers will be used to transport the siRNA-doxorubicin cocktail. The dendrimer system efficiently inhibits gene expression and slows the growth of glioblastoma cells. Coating MSNs with pepsin- and amine-terminated dendrimers have been used to co-deliver MDR-targeted siRNA and doxorubicin [132]. HepG2 drug-resistant human liver cancer cells are given both doxorubicin and siRNA-P-gp at the same time. Micelles' antitumor activity was found to be significantly boosted in HepG2/ADM cells after P-gp downregulation. After 24 hours after injection, nearly all micelles have accumulated in the tumor area, and the co-delivery method significantly restricts tumor growth as a result of synergistic effects [133]. By inhibiting mitotic spindle formation and inducing cell death, Se nanoparticles supported by double hydroxide nanoparticles suppress cell growth by halting the cell cycle at the G2/M phase. These vectors show a potent gene-silencing impact, downregulating P-gp expression and reversing multi-drug resistance in breast cancer cell lines. Nanoscale core-shell coordination polymer nanoparticles loaded with short interfering RNAs (siRNAs) targeting MDR genes improve synergistic therapeutic advantages of cisplatin and overcome MDR in ovarian cancer cell lines and mouse xenograft models [134].

The MDR gene ABCB1 encodes the membrane-bound drug transporter P-gp, which seems to be the fundamental driving force underlying drug resistance. More and more cancer models are using the CRISPR/Cas9 system as a state-of-the-art genome editing technique for overcoming MDR. After a single-guide RNA (sgRNA) recognizes the protospacer neighboring motif downstream of target DNA, Cas9 is utilized as a nuclease to cause a DSB in a particular region. The Cas nuclease can only be directed to the proper spot in the genome by a single-guide RNA (sgRNA) that has already found the target DNA sequence. After the CRISPR/Cas9 system creates a DSB, two error-prone processes, nonhomologous end joining and homologous directed repair, begin repairing DNA, resulting in an insertion or deletion mutation at the target spot. CRISPR/Cas9 has recently been shown to be a powerful gene editing technology, with the ability to silence ABCB1 and bring cancer cells back to their original level of sensitivity to normal therapy. Adeno-associated viruses are used as the vector for delivery, which is the system's main drawback. Multiple strategies for delivering nanoparticles to the affected area have been devised. One such instrument is a cationic polymer-coated gold nanoparticle that facilitates endosomal escape [135].

3.7 Methods of Physical Intervention to Treat MDR

Multiple chemotherapeutic agents have been shown to enter cancer cells successfully through the use of physical methods such as thermal therapy, ultrasonic therapy, and photodynamic therapy. Exogenous heat stress in the range of 41 to 47 degrees Celsius is applied in hyperthermia, also known as thermal therapy [136]. When used in conjunction with other primary therapies, it is well known for significantly increasing the therapeutic efficacy of those therapies [137]. The critical temperature at which the thermosensitive nanocarrier reaches its solution state in water is lower. For instance, the nanocarrier is water-soluble at temperatures below 37 degrees Celsius but is insoluble at higher temperatures, where a conformational shift occurs in the direction of drug release [138]. Therefore, this method is employed as a supplementary treatment to enhance the dispersal of a large number of nanocarriers. Hyperthermia has been linked to a variety of effects, such as the direct killing of tumor cells through denaturing proteins and DNA aggregation and cross-linking, the activation of apoptotic pathways, the alteration of cell cycle regulatory signaling pathways, the alteration of the tumor microenvironment, the activation of heat shock proteins, the induction of the immune response, and the alteration of blood flow, oxygen and nutrient distribution to the tumor. More and more researchers are documenting similar findings [139–142]. The expression levels of MDR-associated proteins are downregulated when BT-474 cells are treated with both magnetic nanoparticles and mitomycin-C. Nonetheless, hyperthermia's consequences are exacerbated. Hyperthermia is able to overcome MDR in many malignancies because it increases drug absorption, induces apoptosis, amplifies drug cytotoxicity, and inactivates drug detoxification systems, all of which are actions mediated by increased intracellular heat [143].

Several clinical investigations have explored the possibility that ultrasonic therapy might improve the effectiveness of treatment against cancer cells. This approach has been used as a hyperthermia-inducing drug in the direct treatment of malignancies and as an adjuvant therapy to boost therapeutic effectiveness when paired with chemotherapeutics. In addition to reversing MDR, ultrasound therapy improves drug delivery by increasing drug diffusion, drug release from nanocarriers, and cellular accumulation of therapeutic agents. Ultrasound is used to transport nanocarriers to the site of cancer, where it triggers nanocarriers to disassemble and release their cargo (usually a drug). Deng *et al.* used doxorubicin–liposome–microbubble complexes in combination with ultrasound to combat the MDR phenotype in resistant human breast cancer MCF-7 cells. They found that when they subjected resistant cells to doxorubicin–liposome–microbubble complexes, ROS levels rose, DNA damage increased, and P-glycoprotein expression decreased. Using a heater assembly of polymeric micelles and liposomes, can make ultrasound-responsive nanobubbles for the treatment of hepatocellular carcinoma. These paclitaxel and siRNA-preserving nanobubbles have been developed. By applying a low-frequency ultrasonic force from the outside, author was able to successfully co-deliver siRNA and paclitaxel to the interior of tumors. The antiapoptosis elicited by paclitaxel treatment in HepG2 cells is thus efficiently suppressed by the Bcl-2 siRNA that is co-delivered throughout chemotherapy [144]. Apoptosis is triggered in HepG2 cells after treatment with paclitaxel, proving this. It has been hypothesized that photodynamic therapy (PDT) can be used to avoid cancer MDR and even resensitize resistant cells to standard therapies due to the damage caused to the tumor cell and the microenvironment by PDT. This is because PDT is an innovative method with significant potential for use in cancer treatment. Light, oxygen, and safe medication to use as a photosensitizer are the three most important components of PDT for inducing photocytotoxicity. Photosensitizers used in photodynamic therapy (PDT) are exposed to light in the 600–800 nm range, which triggers the release of cytotoxic molecular species like reactive oxygen species (ROS) that kill cancer cells. PDT assists in the reversal of MDR by activation of cell death pathways, degradation of proteins responsible for drug resistance, and enhanced drug delivery.

3.8 Conclusion

Clinically, MDR is quite common in the context of cancer treatment, and it necessitates special attention. Without overcoming drug resistance in tumor cells, conventional cancer treatment cannot achieve a complete cure. Increasing the chemotherapeutic dose, turning off genes associated with MDR, and creating inhibitors for ABC transporters are all examples of these approaches. New opportunities have arisen as a result of recent progress in the development of novel approaches in this field. Some of the novel approaches discussed in this article include the use of nanocarriers, RNAi therapy, physical methods, and natural substances. Literature showed that combining RNAi and nanoparticles to create effective medication combinations is much simpler than previous methods. The greatest possible effect may result from this. Combination therapies that use nanocarriers in conjunction with chemotherapeutics or RNA interference are therefore among the most promising methods for combating the rising problem of drug resistance. But there are a lot of issues to solve before the topic can be considered mainstream. One of the biggest obstacles is the high level of specialization required for these treatments. Overcoming MDR without harming normal cells will need the development of novel techniques, such as nanocarriers and RNAi therapy. They will be put to use in the process of delivering drugs to cancer cells in need of treatment. Before these novel drugs can be used in clinical settings, more research is needed to confirm their safety and selectivity.

References

1. Siegel, R.L., Miller, K.D., Jemal, A., Cancer statistics. *CA-Cancer J. Clin.*, 70, 7–30, 2020.
2. Goodman, L.S., Wintrobe, M.M., Dameshek, W., Goodman, M.J., Gilman, A., McLennan, M.T., Use of methyl-bis(beta-chloroethyl)amine hydrochloride and tris(beta-chloroethyl)amine hydrochloride for hodgkin's disease, lymphosarcoma, leukemia and certain allied and miscellaneous disorders. *J. Am. Med. Assoc.*, 132, 126–32, 1946.
3. Chen, X., Lu, P., Wang, D., Yang, S., Wu, Y., Shen, H.-Y. *et al.*, The role of miRNAs in drug resistance and prognosis of breast cancer formalin-fixed paraffin-embedded tissues. *Gene*, 595, 221–6, 2016.
4. Han, J., Sun, W., Liu, R., Zhou, Z., Zhang, H., Chen, X. *et al.*, Plasma exosomal miRNA expression profile as oxaliplatin-based chemoresistant biomarkers in colorectal adenocarcinoma. *Front. Oncol.*, 10, 1495, 2020.
5. Chen, Y., Liu, L., Li, J., Du, Y., Wang, J., Liu, J., Effects of long noncoding RNA (linc-VLDLR) existing in extracellular vesicles on the occurrence and multidrug resistance of esophageal cancer cells. *Pathol. Res. Pract.*, 215, 470–7, 2019.
6. Jin, K.-T., Lu, Z.-B., Lv, J.-Q., Zhang, J.-G., The role of long non-coding RNAs in mediating chemoresistance by modulating autophagy in cancer. *RNA Biol.*, 17, 1727–40, 2020.
7. Chen, C.J., Chin, J.E., Ueda, K., Clark, D.P., Pastan, I., Gottesman, M.M. *et al.*, Internal duplication and homology with bacterial transport proteins in the Mdr1 (P-glycoprotein) gene from multi-drug-resistant human cells. *Cell*, 47, 381–9, 1986.
8. Endicott, J.A. and Ling, V., The biochemistry of P-glycoprotein-mediated multi-drug resistance. *Annu. Rev. Biochem.*, 58, 137–71, 1989.

9. Ernest, S., Rajaraman, S., Megyesi, J., Bello-Reuss, E.N., Expression of MDR1 (multi-drug resistance) gene and its protein in normal human kidney. *Nephron*, 77, 284–9, 1997.
10. Schinkel, A.H., Roelofs, M.E.M., Borst, P., Characterization of the human MDR3 P-glycoprotein and its recognition by P-glycoprotein-specific monoclonal antibodies. *Cancer Res.*, 51, 2628–35, 1991.
11. Ueda, K., Cardarelli, C., Gottesman, M.M., Pastan, T., Expression of a full-length cDNA for the human "Mdr1" gene confers resistance to colchicine, doxorubicin, and vinblastine. *Proc. Natl. Acad. Sci. U.S.A.*, 84, 3004–8, 1987.
12. Kalra, R., Jones, A., Kirk, J., Adams, G.E., Stratford, I.J., The effect of hypoxia on acquired drug resistance and response to epidermal growth factor in chinese hamster lung fibroblasts and human breast-cancer cells *in vitro*. *Int. J. Cancer*, 54, 650–5, 1993.
13. Liang, B.C., Effects of hypoxia on drug resistance phenotype and genotype in human glioma cell lines. *J. Neurooncol.*, 29, 149–55, 1996.
14. Datta, S., Choudhury, D., Das, A., Mukherjee, D.D., Dasgupta, M., Bandopadhyay, S. *et al.*, Autophagy inhibition with chloroquine reverts paclitaxel resistance and attenuates metastatic potential in human nonsmall lung adenocarcinoma A549 cells via ROS mediated modulation of β-catenin pathway. *Apoptosis*, 24, 414–33, 2019.
15. Fu, X.-T., Song, K., Zhou, J., Shi, Y.-H., Liu, W.-R., Shi, G.-M. *et al.*, Tumor-associated macrophages modulate resistance to oxaliplatin via inducing autophagy in hepatocellular carcinoma. *Cancer Cell Int.*, 19, 1–11, 2019.
16. Cancer, Available at: https://www.who.int/health-topics/cancer#tab=tab (Accessed April 22, 2022).
17. Cheung-Ong, K., Giaever, G., Nislow, C., DNA-damaging agents in cancer chemotherapy: Serendipity and chemical biology. *Chem. Biol.*, 20, 648–59, 2013.
18. Mansoori, B., Mohammadi, A., Davudian, S., Shirjang, S., Baradaran, B., The different mechanisms of cancer drug resistance: A brief review. *Adv. Pharm. Bull.*, 7, 339–48, 2017.
19. ErzaMclendzZhong, L., Li, Y., Xiong, L., Wang, W., Wu, M., Yuan, T. *et al.*, Small molecules in targeted cancer therapy: Advances, challenges, and future perspectives. *Signal Transduction Targeting Ther.*, 6, 201, 2021.
20. Pucci, C., Martinelli, C., Ciofani, G., Innovative approaches for cancer treatment: Current perspectives and new challenges. *Ecancermedicalscience*, 13, 961, 2019.
21. Choudhari, A.S., Mandave, P.C., Deshpande, M., Ranjekar, P., Prakash, O., Phytochemicals in cancer treatment: From preclinical studies to clinical practice. *Front. Pharmacol.*, 10, 4–6, 2020.
22. Uramoto, H. and Tanaka, F., Recurrence after surgery in patients with NSCLC. *Transl. Lung Cancer Res.*, 3, 242–9, 2014.

23. Castells, M., Thibault, B., Delord, J.P., Couderc, B., Implication of tumor microenvironment in chemoresistance: Tumor-associated stromal cells protect tumor cells from cell death. *Int. J. Mol. Sci.*, 13, 9545–75, 2012.
24. O'Connor, D., Sibson, K., Caswell, M., Connor, P., Cummins, M., Mitchell, C. *et al.*, Early UK experience in the use of clofarabine in the treatment of relapsed and refractory paediatric acute lymphoblastic leukaemia. *Br. J. Haematol.*, 154, 482–5, 2011.
25. Umar, A., Cancer immunoprevention: A new approach to intercept cancer early. *Cancer Prev. Res.*, 7, 1067–71, 2014.
26. Finn, O.J. and Beatty, P.L., Cancer immunoprevention. *Curr. Opin. Immunol.*, 39, 52–8, 2016.
27. Roseblade, A., Luk, F., Ung, A., Bebawy, M., Targeting microparticle biogenesis: A novel approach to the circumvention of cancer multi-drug resistance. *Curr. Cancer Drug Targets*, 15, 205–14, 2015.
28. Kapse-Mistry, S., Govender, T., Srivastava, R., Yergeri, M., Nanodrug delivery in reversing multi-drug resistance in cancer cells. *Front. Pharmacol.*, 5, 159, 2014.
29. Norouzi-Barough, L., Sarookhani, M., Salehi, R., Sharifi, M., Moghbelinejad, S., CRISPR/Cas9, a new approach to successful knockdown of ABCB1/P-glycoprotein and reversal of chemosensitivity in human epithelial ovarian cancer cell line. *Iran. J. Basic Med. Sci.*, 21, 181, 2018.
30. Zahreddine, H. and Borden, K.L.B., Mechanisms and insights into drug resistance in cancer. *Front. Pharmacol.*, 4, 28, 2013.
31. Zhao, J., Shi, L., Ji, M., Wu, J., Wu, C., The combination of systemic chemotherapy and local treatment may improve the survival of patients with unresectable metastatic colorectal cancer. *Mol. Clin. Oncol.*, 6, 856–60, 2017.
32. Sampath, D., Cortes, J., Estrov, Z., Du, M., Shi, Z., Andreeff, M. *et al.*, Pharmacodynamics of cytarabine alone and in combination with 7-hydroxystaurosporine (UCN-01) in AML blasts *in vitro and* during a clinical trial. *Blood*, 107, 2517–24, 2006.
33. Xue, M., Cheng, J., Zhao, J., Zhang, S., Jian, J., Qiao, Y. *et al.*, Outcomes of 219 chronic myeloid leukaemia patients with additional chromosomal abnormalities and/or tyrosine kinase domain mutations. *Int. J. Lab. Hematol.*, 41, 1–8, 2018.
34. Yeldag, A. and del Rio Hernandez, A., Chemoresistance and the self-maintaining tumor microenvironment. *Cancers*, 10, 471, 2018.
35. Gupta, P.B., Fillmore, C.M., Jiang, G., Shapira, S.D., Tao, K., Kuperwasser, C. *et al.*, Stochastic state transitions give rise to phenotypic equilibrium in populations of cancer cells. *Cell*, 146, 633–44, 2011.
36. Arora, V.K., Schenkein, E., Murali, R., Subudhi, S.K., Wongvipat, J., Balbas, M.D. *et al.*, Glucocorticoid receptor confers resistance to antiandrogens by bypassing androgen receptor blockade. *Cell*, 155, 1309–22, 2013.

37. Benner, S.E., Wahl, G.M., von Hoff, D.D., Double minute chromosomes and homogeneously staining regions in tumors taken directly from patients versus in human tumor cell lines. *Anticancer Drugs*, 2, 11–25, 1991.
38. Li, Z.W. and Dalton, W.S., Tumor microenvironment and drug resistance in hematologic malignancies. *Blood Rev.*, 20, 333–42, 2006.
39. Gottesman, M.M., Mechanisms of cancer drug resistance. *Annu. Rev. Med.*, 53, 615–27, 2002.
40. Wang, Z., Shen, Z., Li, Z., Duan, J., Fu, S., Liu, Z. *et al.*, Activation of the BMP-BMPR pathway conferred resistance to EGFR-TKIs in lung squamous cell carcinoma patients with EGFR mutations. *Proc. Natl. Acad. Sci.*, 1–6, 9990–5, 2015.
41. Wang, X., Zhang, H., Chen, X., Drug resistance and combating drug resistance in cancer. *Cancer Drug Resist. PNAS U.S.A.*, 2, 141, 2019.
42. Meacham, C.E. and Morrison, S.J., Tumor heterogeneity and cancer cell plasticity. *Nature*, 501, 328, 2013, doi: 10.1038/NATURE12624.
43. Huang, D., Duan, H., Huang, H., Tong, X., Han, Y., Ru, G. *et al.*, Cisplatin resistance in gastric cancer cells is associated with HER2 upregulation-induced epithelial-mesenchymal transition. *Sci. Rep.*, 6, 1–12, 2016.
44. Kurrey, N.K., Jalgaonkar, S.P., Joglekar, A.V., Ghanate, A.D., Chaskar, P.D., Doiphode, R.Y. *et al.*, Snail and slug mediate radioresistance and chemoresistance by antagonizing P53-mediated apoptosis and acquiring a stem-like phenotype in ovarian cancer cells. *Stem Cells*, 27, 2059–68, 2009.
45. Kreso, A., Brien, C.A.O., Vzn Galen, P., Gan, O., Notta, F., Variable clonal repopulation dynamics influence chemotherapy response in colorectal cancer resp, in: *Variable Clonal Repopulation Dynamics Influence*, p. 1227670, American Association for the Advancement of Science, Washington, D.C., United States, 2012, Available at: http://www.sciencemag.org/content/early/2012/12/12/science.1227670.
46. Nathanson, D.A., Gini, B., Mottahedeh, J., Visnyei, K., Koga, T., Gomez, G. *et al.*, Targeted therapy resistance mediated by dynamic regulation of extrachromosomal mutant EGFR DNA. *Sci. (1979)*, 343, 72–6, 2014.
47. Gatenby, R.A., Gillies, R.J., Brown, J.S., The evolutionary dynamics of cancer prevention. *Nat. Rev. Cancer*, 10, 526–7, 2010.
48. Junttila, M.R. and De Sauvage, F.J., Influence of tumour micro-environment heterogeneity on therapeutic response. *Nature*, 501, 346–54, 2013.
49. Ding, L., Ley, T.J., Larson, D.E., Miller, C.A., Koboldt, D.C., Welch, J.S. *et al.*, Clonal evolution in relapsed acute myeloid leukaemia revealed by whole-genome sequencing. *Nature*, 481, 506–10, 2012.
50. Quintás-Cardama, A., Kantarjian, H.M., Cortes, J.E., Mechanisms of primary and secondary resistance to imatinib in chronic myeloid leukemia. *Cancer Control*, 16, 122–31, 2009.
51. Kimura, S., Toshihiko, A., Kojima, K., BCR-ABL point mutations and TKI treatment in CML patients. *J. Hematol. Transfus.*, 17, 113–23, 1963.

52. Challagundla, K.B., Wise, P.M., Neviani, P., Chava, H., Murtadha, M., Xu, T. *et al.*, Exosome-mediated transfer of microRNAs within the tumor microenvironment and neuroblastoma resistance to chemotherapy. *J. Natl. Cancer Inst.*, 107, 1–13, 2015.
53. di Virgilio, F., Sarti, A.C., Falzoni, S., de Marchi, E., Adinolfi, E., Extracellular ATP and P2 purinergic signalling in the tumour microenvironment. *Nat. Rev. Cancer*, 18, 601–18, 2018.
54. Wang, X., Li, Y., Qian, Y., Cao, Y., Shriwas, P., Extracellular ATP , as an energy and phosphorylating molecule, induces different types of drug resistances in cancer cells through ATP internalization and intracellular ATP level increase. *Oncotarget*, 8, 87860–77, 2017.
55. Pearce, E.L., Poffenberger, M.C., Chang, C.H., Jones, R.G., Fueling immunity: Insights into metabolism and lymphocyte function. *Sci. (1979)*, 342, 1242454, 2013.
56. Qian, Y., Wang, X., Liu, Y., Li, Y., Colvin, R.A., Tong, L. *et al.*, Extracellular ATP is internalized by macropinocytosis and induces intracellular ATP increase and drug resistance in cancer cells. *Cancer Lett.*, 351, 242–51, 2014.
57. Schneider, V., Krieger, M.L., Bendas, G., Jaehde, U., Kalayda, G.V., Contribution of intracellular ATP to cisplatin resistance of tumor cells. *J. Biol. Inorg. Chem.*, 18, 165–74, 2013.
58. Koppenol, W.H., Bounds, P.L., Dang, C.V., Otto warburg's contributions to current concepts of cancer metabolism. *Nat. Rev. Cancer*, 11, 325–37, 2011.
59. Zhou, Y., Tozzi, F., Chen, J., Fan, F., Xia, L., Wang, J. *et al.*, Intracellular ATP levels are a pivotal determinant of chemoresistance in colon cancer cells. *Cancer Res.*, 72, 304–15, 2012.
60. Rees, D.C., Johnson, E., Lewinson, O., ABC transporters: The power to change. *Nat. Rev. Mol. Cell Biol.*, 10, 218–27, 2009.
61. Reis, R. and Moraes, I., Structural biology and structure–function relationships of membrane proteins. *Biochem. Soc. Trans.*, 47, 47–61, 2019.
62. ter Beek, J., Guskov, A., Slotboom, D.J., Structural diversity of ABC transporters. *J. Gen. Physiol.*, 143, 419–35, 2014.
63. Townsend, D.M. and Tew, K.D., The role of glutathione-s-transferase in anti-cancer drug resistance. *Oncogene*, 22, 7369–75, 2003.
64. Cumming, R.C., Lightfoot, J., Beard, K., Youssoufian, H., O'brien, P.J., Buchwald, M., Fanconi anemia group c protein prevents apoptosis in hematopoietic cells through redox regulation of GSTP1. *Nat. Med.*, 7, 814–20, 2001.
65. Manolitsas, T.P., Englefield, P., Eccles, D.M., Campbell, I.G., No association of a 306-Bp insertion polymorphism in the progesterone receptor gene with ovarian and breast cancer. *Br. J. Cancer*, 75, 1398–9, 1997.
66. Di Virgilio, F. and Adinolfi, E., Extracellular purines, purinergic receptors and tumor growth. *Oncogene*, 36, 293–303, 2017, doi: 10.1038/onc.2016.206.
67. Burnstock, G. and Di Virgilio, F., Purinergic signalling and cancer. *Purinergic Signalling*, 9, 491–540, 2013.

68. Salvestrini, V., Zini, R., Rossi, L., Gulinelli, S., Manfredini, R., Bianchi, E. *et al.*, Purinergic signaling inhibits human acute myeloblastic leukemia cell proliferation, migration, and engraftment in immunodeficient mice. *Blood*, 119, 217–26, 2012.
69. Zandvliet, M. and Teske, E., Mechanisms of drug resistance in veterinary oncology. *Vet. Sci.*, 2, 150–84, 2015.
70. Sahoo, S., Aurich, M.K., Jonsson, J.J., Thiele, I., Membrane transporters in a human genome-scale metabolic knowledgebase and their implications for disease. *Front. Physiol.*, 5, 1–24, 2014.
71. Spreckelmeyer, S., Orvig, C., Casini, A., Cellular transport mechanisms of cytotoxic metallodrugs: An overview beyond cisplatin. *Molecules*, 19, 15584–610, 2014.
72. Goldman, I.D., Membrane transport of chemotherapeutics and drug resistance: Beyond the ABC family of exporters to the role of carrier-mediated processes. *Clin. Cancer Res.*, 8, 4–6, 2002.
73. Al-Anazi, K.A., Eltayeb, K.I., Bakr, M., Al-Mohareb, F.I., Methotrexate-induced acute leukemia: Report of three cases and review of the literature. *Clin. Med. Case Rep.*, 2, 43, 2009.
74. Kyung, T.O., Hye JB, A.H.L., Young, T.O., Yu, S.Y., Eun, S.L., The reversal of drug-resistance in tumors using a drug-carrying nanoparticular system. *Int. J. Mol. Sci.*, 10, 3776–92, 2009.
75. Hu, X. and Zhang, Z., Understanding the genetic mechanisms of cancer drug resistance using genomic approaches. *Trends Genet.*, 32, 127–37, 2016.
76. Longo-Sorbello, G.S. and Bertino, J.R., Current understanding of methotrexate pharmacology and efficacy in acute leukemias. Use of newer antifolates in clinical trials. *Haematologica*, 86, 121–7, 2001.
77. Juliano, R.L. and Ling, V., A surface glycoprotein modulating drug permeability in chinese hamster ovary cell mutants. *BBA – Biomembranes*, 455, 152–62, 1976.
78. Cole, S.P.C., Bhardwaj, G., Gerlach, J.H., Mackie, J.E., Grant, C.E., Almquist, K.C. *et al.*, Overexpression of a transporter gene in a multi-drug-resistant human lung cancer cell line. *Science*, 258, 1650–4, 1992.
79. Austin Doyle, L., Yang, W., Abruzzo, L.V., Krogmann, T., Gao, Y., Rishi, A.K. *et al.*, A multi-drug resistance transporter from human MCF-7 breast cancer cells. *Proc. Natl. Acad. Sci. U.S.A.*, 95, 15665–70, 1998.
80. Ku, E., Bogman, K., Peyer, A., To, M., HMG-CoA reductase inhibitors and P-glycoprotein modulation. *Br. J. Pharmacol.*, 132, 1183–92, 2001.
81. Awad, M.M., Katayama, R., McTigue, M., Liu, W., Deng, Y.-L., Brooun, A. *et al.*, Acquired resistance to crizotinib from a mutation in CD74 – ros1. *N. Engl. J. Med.*, 368, 2395–401, 2013.
82. Montagut, C., Dalmases, A., Bellosillo, B., Crespo, M., Pairet, S., Iglesias, M. *et al.*, Identification of a mutation in the extracellular domain of the epidermal growth factor receptor conferring cetuximab resistance in colorectal cancer. *Nat. Med.*, 18, 221–3, 2012.

83. Engelman, J.A., Mukohara, T., Zejnullahu, K., Lifshits, E., Borrás, A.M., Gale, C.M. *et al.*, Allelic dilution obscures detection of a biologically significant resistance mutation in EGFR-amplified lung cancer. *J. Clin. Invest.*, 116, 2695–706, 2006.
84. Niederst, M.J. and Engelman, J.A., Bypass mechanisms of resistance to receptor tyrosine kinase inhibition in lung cancer. *Sci. Signaling*, 6, 1–7, 2013.
85. Lee, H.J., Zhuang, G., Cao, Y., Du, P., Kim, H.J., Settleman, J., Drug resistance via feedback activation of stat3 in oncogene-addicted cancer cells. *Cancer Cell*, 26, 207–21, 2014.
86. Zhang, Y.-W., Zheng, Y., Wang, J., Lu, X., Wang, Z., Chen, L., Integrated analysis of DNA methylation and mRNA expression profiling reveals candidate genes associated with cisplatin resistance in non-small cell lung cancer. *Epigenetics*, 9, 37–41, 2014.
87. Konieczkowski, D.J., Johannessen, C.M., Abudayyeh, O., Kim, J.W., Cooper, Z.A., Piris, A. *et al.*, A melanoma cell state distinction influences sensitivity to MAPK pathway inhibitors. *Cancer Discovery*, 4, 816–27, 2014.
88. Straussman, R., Morikawa, T., Shee, K., Barzily-Rokni, M., Qian, Z.R., Du, J. *et al.*, Tumour micro-environment elicits innate resistance to RAF inhibitors through HGF secretion. *Nature*, 487, 500–4, 2012.
89. Hirata, E., Girotti, M.R., Viros, A., Hooper, S., Spencer-Dene, B., Matsuda, M. *et al.*, Intravital imaging reveals how BRAF inhibition generates drug-tolerant microenvironments with high integrin β1/FAK signaling. *Cancer Cell*, 27, 574–88, 2015.
90. Sharma, S.V., Lee, D.Y., Li, B., Quinlan, M.P., Takahashi, F., Maheswaran, S. *et al.*, A chromatin-mediated reversible drug-tolerant state in cancer cell subpopulations. *Cell*, 141, 69–80, 2010.
91. Zeller, C., Dai, W., Steele, N.L., Siddiq, A., Walley, A.J., Rizzo, S. *et al.*, Candidate DNA methylation drivers of acquired cisplatin resistance in ovarian cancer identified by methylome and expression profiling. *Oncogene*, 31, 4567–76, 2012.
92. Bauer, S., Hilger, R.A., Mühlenberg, T., Grabellus, F., Nagarajah, J., Hoiczyk, M. *et al.*, Phase I study of panobinostat and imatinib in patients with treatment-refractory metastatic gastrointestinal stromal tumors. *Br. J. Cancer*, 110, 1155–62, 2014.
93. Glasspool, R.M., Brown, R., Gore, M.E., Rustin, G.J.S., McNeish, I.A., Wilson, R.H. *et al.*, A randomised, phase II trial of the DNA-hypomethylating agent 5-aza-2′-deoxycytidine (decitabine) in combination with carboplatin vs carboplatin alone in patients with recurrent, partially platinum-sensitive ovarian cancer. *Br. J. Cancer*, 110, 1923–9, 2014.
94. Tulsyan, S., Mittal, R.D., Mittal, B., The effect of ABCB1 polymorphisms on the outcome of breast cancer treatment. *Pharmacogenomics Pers. Med.*, 9, 47, 2016.
95. Yasuhisa, K., Shin-ya, M., Michinori, M., Kazumitsu, U., Mechanism of multidrug recognition by MDR1/ABCB1. *Cancer Sci.*, 98, 1303–10, 2007.

96. Kurz, E.U., Cole, S.P.C., Deeley, R.G., Identification of DNA-protein interactions in the 5′ flanking and 5′ untranslated regions of the human multidrug resistance protein (MRP1) gene: Evaluation of a putative antioxidant response element/AP-1 binding site. *Biochem. Biophys. Res. Commun.*, 285, 981–90, 2001.
97. Dean, M., Hamon, Y., Chimini, G., The human ATP-binding cassette (ABC) transporter superfamily. *J. Lipid Res.*, 42, 1007–17, 2001.
98. Jedlitschky, G., Hoffmann, U., Kroemer, H.K., Structure and function of the MRP2 (ABCC2) protein and its role in drug disposition. *Expert Opin. Drug Metab. Toxicol.*, 2, 351–66, 2006.
99. Yamasaki, M., Makino, T., Masuzawa, T., Kurokawa, Y., Miyata, H., Takiguchi, S. *et al.*, Role of multi-drug resistance protein 2 (MRP2) in chemoresistance and clinical outcome in oesophageal squamous cell carcinoma. *Br. J. Cancer*, 104, 707–13, 2011.
100. Lee, J.H., Chen, H.L., Chen, H.L., Ni, Y.H., Hsu, H.Y., Chang, M.H., Neonatal Dubin-Johnson syndrome: Long-term follow-up and MRP2 mutations study. *Pediatr. Res.*, 59, 584–9, 2006.
101. Hou, Y., Zhu, Q., Li, Z., Peng, Y., Yu, X., Yuan, B. *et al.*, The FOXM1-ABCC5 axis contributes to paclitaxel resistance in nasopharyngeal carcinoma cells. *Cell Death Dis.*, 8, e2659–11, 2017.
102. Lal, S., Sutiman, N., Ooi, L.L., Wong, Z.W., Wong, N.S., Ang, P.C.S. *et al.*, Pharmacogenetics of ABCB5, ABCC5 and RLIP76 and doxorubicin pharmacokinetics in asian breast cancer patients. *Pharmacogenomics J.*, 17, 337–43, 2017.
103. Mo, W. and Zhang, J.T., Human ABCG2: Structure, function, and its role in multi-drug resistance. *Int. J. Biochem. Mol. Biol.*, 3, 1, 2012.
104. Human gene ABCG2 (ENST00000650821.1) from GENCODE V39, Available at: https://genome.ucsc.edu/cgi-bin/hgGene?db=hg38&hgg_gene=ABCG2 (Accessed May 5, 2022).
105. Abcg2 ATP binding cassette subfamily G member 2 (Junior blood group) [Mus musculus (house mouse)], Gene - NCBI, Available at: https://www.ncbi.nlm.nih.gov/gene?Db=gene&Cmd=DetailsSearch&Term=26357 (Accessed May 5, 2022).
106. García-Aranda, M., Pérez-Ruiz, E., Redondo, M., Bcl-2 inhibition to overcome resistance to chemo-and immunotherapy. *Int. J. Mol. Sci.*, 19, 3950, 2018.
107. Marie Hardwick, J. and Soane, L., Multiple functions of BCL-2 family proteins. *Cold Spring Harb. Perspect. Biol.*, 5, a008722, 2013.
108. Qu, Q., Mao, Y., Fei, X.C., Shen, K.W., The impact of androgen receptor expression on breast cancer survival: A retrospective study and meta-analysis. *PLoS One*, 8, 1–8, 2013.
109. Sigismund, S., Avanzato, D., Lanzetti, L., Emerging functions of the EGFR in cancer. *Mol. Oncol.*, 12, 3–20, 2018.

110. Hientz, K., Mohr, A., Bhakta-Guha, D., Efferth, T., The role of P53 in cancer drug resistance and targeted chemotherapy. *Oncotarget*, 8, 8921–46, 2017.
111. Zhou, X., Hao, Q., Lu, H., Mutant P53 in cancer therapy – the barrier or the path. *J. Mol. Cell Biol.*, 11, 293–305, 2019.
112. Ohata, Y., Shimada, S., Akiyama, Y., Mogushi, K., Nakao, K., Satoshi Matsumura, S. *et al.*, Acquired resistance with epigenetic alterations under long-term anti-angiogenic therapy for hepatocellular carcinoma. *Mol. Cancer Ther.*, 16, 6, 1161–1163, 2017.
113. Chen, Q.N., Wei, C.C., Wang, Z.X., Sun, M., Long non-coding RNAs in anti-cancer drug resistance. *Oncotarget*, 8, 1925–36, 2017.
114. Malek, E., Jagannathan, S., Driscoll, J.J., Correlation of long non-coding RNA expression with metastasis, drug resistance and clinical outcome in cancer. *Oncotarget*, 5, 8027–38, 2014.
115. Ghasemi, S., Mozdarani, H., Soleimani, M., The effect of miR-372 on genome instability in MKN-45 cell line. *J. Isfahan Med. Sch.*, 32, 3–8, 2015.
116. Housman, G., Byler, S., Heerboth, S., Lapinska, K., Longacre, M., Snyder, N. *et al.*, Drug resistance in cancer: An overview. *Cancers (Basel)*, 6, 1769–92, 2014.
117. Ghasemi, S., Razmkhah, F., Soleimani, M., The role of epigenetics in cancer drug resistance. *J. Kerman Univ. Med. Sci.*, 24, 250–8, 2017.
118. Choi, S.W. and Friso, S., Epigenetics: A new bridge between nutrition and health. *Adv. Nutr.*, 1, 8–16, 2010.
119. Fojo, A., Hamilton, T.C., Young, R.C., Ozols, R.F., Multi-drug resistance in ovarian cancer. *Cancer*, 60, 2075–80, 1987.
120. Gong, J., Jaiswal, R., Mathys, J.-M., Combes, V., Grau, G.E.R., Bebawy, M., Microparticles and their emerging role in cancer multi-drug resistance. *Cancer Treat. Rev.*, 38, 226–34, 2012.
121. Baguley, B.C., Multi-drug resistance in cancer, in: *Multi-Drug Resistance in Cancer*, J. Zhou (Ed.), pp. 1–14, Humana Press, Totowa, NJ, 2010.
122. An, X., Sarmiento, C., Tan, T., Zhu, H., Regulation of multi-drug resistance by microRNAs in anti-cancer therapy. *Acta Pharm. Sin. B*, 7, 38–51, 2017.
123. Moitra, K., Overcoming multi-drug resistance in cancer stem cells. *Biomed. Res. Int.*, 2015, 635745, 2015.
124. Ho, E.A. and Piquette-Miller, M., Regulation of multi-drug resistance by pro-inflammatory cytokines. *Curr. Cancer Drug Targets*, 6, 295–311, 2006.
125. Xue, Z., Yan, H., Li, J., Liang, S., Cai, X., Chen, X. *et al.*, Identification of cancer stem cells in vincristine preconditioned SGC7901 gastric cancer cell line. *J. Cell. Biochem.*, 113, 302–12, 2012.
126. Sarvi, S., Mackinnon, A.C., Avlonitis, N., Bradley, M., Rintoul, R.C., Rassl, D.M. *et al.*, CD133+ cancer stem-like cells in small cell lung cancer are highly tumorigenic and chemoresistant but sensitive to a novel neuropeptide antagonist. *Cancer Res.*, 74, 1554–65, 2014.
127. Martin, V., Sanchez-Sanchez, A.M., Herrera, F., Gomez-Manzano, C., Fueyo, J., Alvarez-Vega, M.A. *et al.*, Melatonin-induced methylation of the ABCG2/

BCRP promoter as a novel mechanism to overcome multi-drug resistance in brain tumour stem cells. *Br. J. Cancer*, 108, 2005–12, 2013.

128. Cheng, W., Liu, T., Wan, X., Gao, Y., Wang, H., MicroRNA-199a targets CD44 to suppress the tumorigenicity and multi-drug resistance of ovarian cancer-initiating cells. *FEBS J.*, 279, 2047–59, 2012.
129. Wang, F., Li, T., Zhang, B., Li, H., Wu, Q., Yang, L. *et al.*, MicroRNA-19a/B regulates multi-drug resistance in human gastric cancer cells by targeting PTEN. *Biochem. Biophys. Res. Commun.*, 434, 688–94, 2013.
130. Zhang, L., Pickard, K., Jenei, V., Bullock, M.D., Bruce, A., Mitter, R. *et al.*, miR-153 supports colorectal cancer progression *via* pleiotropic effects that enhance invasion and chemotherapeutic resistance. *Cancer Res.*, 73, 6435–47, 2013.
131. Xia, L., Zhang, D., Du, R., Pan, Y., Zhao, L., Sun, S. *et al.*, miR-15b and miR-16 modulate multi-drug resistance by targeting BCL2 in human gastric cancer cells. *Int. J. Cancer*, 123, 372–9, 2008.
132. Shang, Y., Zhang, Z., Liu, Z., Feng, B., Ren, G., Li, K. *et al.*, miR-508-5p regulates multi-drug resistance of gastric cancer by targeting ABCB1 and ZNRD1. *Oncogene*, 33, 3267–76, 2014.
133. Chen, Z., Ma, T., Huang, C., Zhang, L., Lv, X., Xu, T. *et al.*, MiR-27a modulates the MDR1/P-glycoprotein expression by inhibiting FZD7/β-catenin pathway in hepatocellular carcinoma cells. *Cell Signal.*, 25, 2693–701, 2013.
134. Chen, Q., Xia, H.-W., Ge, X.-J., Zhang, Y.-C., Tang, Q.-L., Bi, F., Serum miR-19a predicts resistance to FOLFOX chemotherapy in advanced colorectal cancer cases. *Asian Pac. J. Cancer Prev.*, 14, 7421–6, 2013.
135. Frei, I.I.I.E., Karon, M., Levin, R.H., Freireich, E.J., Taylor, R.J., Hananian, J. *et al.*, The effectiveness of combinations of antileukemic agents in inducing and maintaining remission in children with acute leukemia. *Blood*, 26, 642–56, 1965.
136. Jones, V.S., Huang, R.Y., Chen, L.P., Chen, Z.S., Fu, L., Huang, R.P., Cytokines in cancer drug resistance: Cues to new therapeutic strategies. *Biochim. Biophys. Acta (BBA) – Rev. Cancer*, 1865, 255–65, 2016.
137. Walther, W. and Stein, U., Influence of cytokines Onmdr1 expression in human colon carcinoma cell lines: Increased cytoxicity of MDR relevant drugs. *J. Cancer Res. Clin. Oncol.*, 120, 471–8, 1994, doi: 10.1007/BF01191800.
138. Curiel, T.J., Immunotherapy: A useful strategy to help combat multi-drug resistance. *Drug Resist. Updat.*, 15, 106–13, 2012.
139. Aluigi, M.G., Debernardis, D., Cimoli, G., Ottoboni, C., Parodi, S., Russo, P., Tumor-necrosis-factor and DNA topoisomerase-ii inhibitors in human ovarian-cancer-potential role in chemotherapy. *Int. J. Oncol.*, 7, 461–7, 1995.
140. Mosaffa, F., Kalalinia, F., Parhiz, B.H., Behravan, J., Tumor necrosis factor alpha induces stronger cytotoxicity in ABCG2-overexpressing resistant breast cancer cells compared with their drug-sensitive parental line. *DNA Cell Biol.*, 30, 413–8, 2011.

141. Stein, U., Walther, W., Shoemaker, R.H., Schlag, P.M., IL-2 gene transfer for chemosensitization of multi-drug-resistant human colon carcinoma cells, in: *Gene Therapy of Cancer*, P. Walden, U. Trefzer, W. Sterry, F. Farzaneh, P. Zambon (Eds.), pp. 145–9, Springer US, Boston, MA, 1998.
142. Walther, W., Stein, U., Fichtner, I., Alexander, M., Shoemaker, R.H., Schlag, P.M., Mdr1 promoter-driven tumor necrosis factor-α expression for a chemotherapy-controllable combined *in vivo* gene therapy and chemotherapy of tumors. *Cancer Gene Ther.*, 7, 893–900, 2000.
143. Yu, D., The role of oncogenes in drug resistance. *Cytotechnology*, 27, 283–92, 1998.
144. Croce, C.M., Oncogenes and cancer. Supplementary appendix. *N. Engl. J. Med.*, 358, 502–11, 2008.

4

Natural Products for Clinical Management of Drug Resistant Cancer Cells

Rishabha Malviya*, Arun Kumar Singh and Deepika Yadav

Abstract

Cancers develop chemotherapeutic medication resistance via multi-drug resistance. It is a major cause of chemotherapy failure. This review discusses tumor drug resistance and efforts to find chemicals that interact with multi-drug-resistant cells. This information can help with retrospective investigations and identifying novel drug development prospects to treat multi-drug-resistant cell types.

Keywords: Natural products, multi-drug resistance, multi-drug resistance modulators, herbal components, resistance mechanism

4.1 Introduction

MDR complicates the treatment of infectious illnesses and malignancies. Current cancer therapies frequently fail at some point. Many tumors grow chemoresistant, making them untreatable. 90% of metastatic cancer patients are MDR-resistant [1]. Cancers of the breast, intestine, lung, and ovaries are impacted by multi-drug resistance. Because tumors can take on so many different forms, it is not unusual for drug-sensitive and drug-resistant cells to coexist within the same tumor. A tumor's drug-sensitive cells will be eliminated by early anti-cancer therapy, but a significant number of resistant cells will remain. Tumors develop resistance to treatment when drug-resistant cells multiply uncontrollably among sensitive ones [2]. Figure 4.1 depicts natural products used in cancer therapy.

**Corresponding author*: rishabhamalviya19@gmail.com

Rishabha Malviya, Arun Kumar Singh and Deepika Yadav. Multi-Drug Resistance in Cancer: Mechanism and Treatment Strategies, (77–86) © 2023 Scrivener Publishing LLC

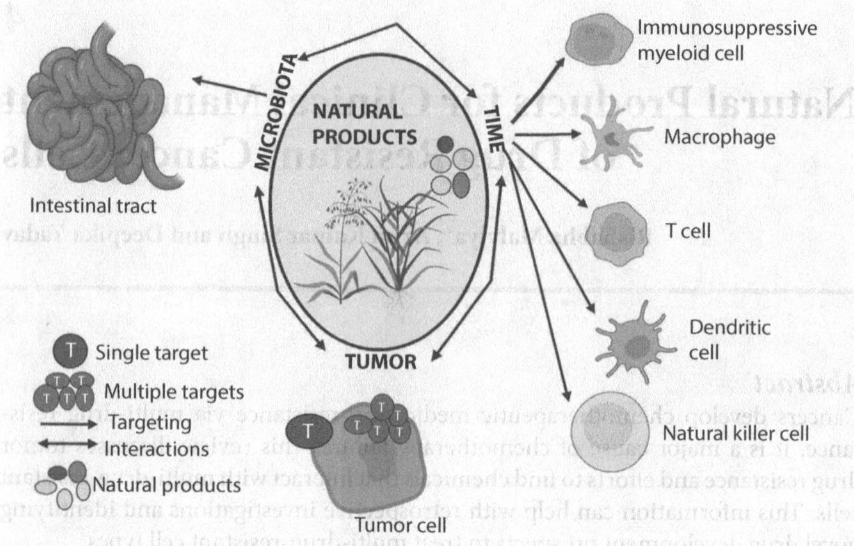

Figure 4.1 Diagrammatic representation of natural products in cancer therapy.

4.2 Resistance Mechanisms

There has been a lot of investigation on the root causes of drug resistance. There are primarily three strategies that cells use to reject medicines. Water-soluble medicines such as cisplatin, foliate antagonists, and nucleoside analogues are less likely to be taken up by cells. One possible explanation for this decline is the increase in the expression of drug transporters like P-glycoprotein. In order to reduce the concentration of anticancer medications below the threshold at which they become cytotoxic, these transporters may export them from the cell. Cytotoxic drugs may lose their toxicity if they cause changes in the cell cycle, improve DNA repair, reduce apoptosis, or alter drug metabolism. The capacity to resist apoptosis is a common feature of human malignancies. An uptick in antiapoptotic molecules or the reduction in function or deficiencies in proapoptotic proteins might, in theory, halt the signaling cascade that leads to cell death. There is evidence linking the mitochondrial surface protein Bcl-2, which suppresses the apoptotic cascade, to the onset and spread of various forms of cancer [3–5]. This molecule blocks the release of apoptosis-inducing cytoplasmic chemicals by inhibiting pore formation in the mitochondrial membrane. Thus, decreased Bcl-2 expression may make tumors more susceptible to antineoplastic medicines and shorten their survival time. Substances that inhibit Bcl-2 have therefore been the subject of substantial research [5–7]. Increased energy-dependent efflux of hydrophobic medications that normally enter cells via diffusion across the plasma membrane is the third mechanism by which drug resistance emerges [2]. As cancer angiogenesis is a growth inhibitor, inherent resistance to antiangiogenic treatment must be high. This novel theory proposes that angiogenic tumors may develop resistance to therapeutic angiogenesis suppression by adapting to the presence of angiogenesis inhibitors [8, 9]. The activation of alternative mechanisms for sustaining tumor growth while the antiangiogenic drug continues to inhibit its specific therapeutic target is a hallmark of evasive resistance [10–12]. In contrast to popular perception, drug resistance is not caused by changes in drug absorption and efflux or mutations in drug target genes.

At least four adaptive mechanisms connected to vascular endothelial growth factor (VEGF) signaling may result in evasive resistance to antiangiogenic treatment. p53 expression was upregulated, alternative proangiogenic signaling pathways were activated or overexpressed in the tumors, and proangiogenic cells were recruited from the patient's bone marrow.

Since the majority of cancer patients pass away after their widespread cancer has become resistant to all current therapies, drug resistance continues to be one of the greatest obstacles in the management of cancer patients.

4.3 Antitumor Plants for Multi-Drug-Resistant Cells

One of humanity's earliest traditions is still widely practiced today: the harvesting and use of plants for medical purposes. Herbal medicine experienced a resurgence in the West at the end of the 20th century as people started to see traditional pharmacopoeias as important sources of accessible treatments and started to believe that natural supplements were safer and more effective than those made from allopathic pharmaceuticals. The vast majority of allopathic pharmaceuticals are derived from plant species, so this recognition is not surprising. Vincristine and vinblastine, two anticancer drugs produced from the vinca plant, were discovered in the 1950s [13]. For this, beginning in the 1960s, the National Cancer Institute in the United States began an extensive sampling operation, primarily in temperate regions. Several chemicals, such as camptothecins and taxanes, with a variety of cytotoxic properties, were discovered as a result of this study. Since the programme ended in 1982, there has been a resurgence of interest in collecting plants and other species from throughout the world, with an emphasis on the subtropical and tropical areas, in order to perform screens of biological activity. As a result, scientists have begun investigating natural compounds to create cutting-edge cancer treatments. While there are many effective treatments for cancer, most cancers eventually develop resistance to at least one of these medications. These constraints have prompted the hunt for novel, efficient chemicals that have no undesirable side effects. This is important since recent studies have shown that natural compounds may serve as MDR modulators. As a result, the researcher know quite a bit about a few natural products. As one example, the cortical material of Simaroubaceae species, known scientifically as quassina, has an extremely bitter taste.

It has been shown that certain quassinoids have cytotoxic and antitumor effects [14, 15]. Although cedronolactone and 14-hydroxychaparrinone are two of the most effective quassinoids [15] for treating lymphocytic leukemia P388 cells, these cells show resistance to a wide range of anticancer therapies. *In vitro* testing of various quanioids revealed high sensitivity in five multi-drug-resistant tumor cell lines (A549, TE-671, HCT-8, KB, and RPMI-7951) and one lymphocytic leukemia cell line (P338). The quasinoids euricomalactone, b-dihydroxyclaineanone, 6-dihydroxylongilactone, and pasakbumina C significantly suppressed the growth of the multi-drug-resistant MCF-7 human breast cancer cell line and the A-549 lung cancer cell line [14]. The amounts of betulinic, oleanolic, and pomolic acids in extracts of *Chrysobalanus icaco* leaves and *Licania tomentosa* fruit were separately assessed. In an erythroleukemic cell line, this particular category of triterpenoids reduced cell proliferation and brought about cell death (K562). "They had a significant impact on Lucena1, a K562 subgroup that is resistant to vincristine and has various drug resistance pathways [15].

Natural compounds may have properties other than cytotoxicity that may be used to combat MDR cells. Some plants have been shown to alter tumor cells' resistance to anticancer medicines [16, 17].

KB-V1 cells, which are MDR human cervical cancer cells with high P-glycoprotein (P-gp) expression, regained sensitivity to colchicine, paclitaxel, and vinblastine after receiving therapy with *Stemona curtisii* root extract [18]. Chemosensitizing properties of the *S. curtisii* extract were shown using the MTT [3-(4,5-dimethythiazol-2-yl)-2,5-diphenyl tetrazolium bromide] assay. According to the specific *in vitro* inhibition of P-gp that *S. curtisii* extract caused, it may help treat multi-drug-resistant cancers by decreasing the efflux of anticancer medicines. To investigate the effects of *Curcuma wenyujin* (C10 and E10) and *Chrysanthemum indicum* fractions on the MDR genotypic and P-gp function in MCF-7/ADR and A549/Taxol cells, *in vitro* experiments were performed (E10). Rhodamine

123 was used to quantify P-gp activity, and MCF-7/ADR cells took up and secreted the dye. Curcumin, an ingredient in *C. wenyujin* C10, has been shown to decrease P-gp expression in MDR cells, with the greatest inhibitory effect seen in MCF7/ADR cells at nontoxic doses. Furthermore, the effects of these three fractions when combined increased the apoptosis that doxorubicin inflicted on MCF-7/ADR cells and counteracted the G2/M arrest that docetaxel imposed on A549/Taxol cells [19].

Fruits, nuts, vegetables, plant-based drinks, traditional Chinese medicine, and herb-based nutritional supplements are all good sources of flavonoids. These chemicals, known as chemosensitizers, target P-gp at its ATP-binding site and its hydrophobic region that interacts with vicinal steroids [20, 21]. Comparing the P-gp activity of the sensitive MCF-7 and the resistant MCF-7/ADR human breast cancer cell lines, Chung *et al.* [22] looked into the effects of various flavonoids. Biochanin A, diadzein, fisetin, morin, naringenin, quercetin, and silymarin were all identified as flavonoids among these plants. Using a sulforhodamine B staining experiment, the author found that the addition of biochanin A and silymarin significantly decreased the IC50 value of the reference drug daunomycin, indicating an increase in cytotoxicity. Silymarin exhibited a similar effect to the P-gp inhibitor verapamil in preventing daunomycin accumulation, but biochanin A had the largest impact. This research shows that adding silymarin to biochanin A improves the effectiveness of chemotherapy drugs [22].

Resveratrol, a flavonoid-like chemical, has been found to kill certain types of tumor cells. It is taken from the skins of several plants, including mulberries and red grapes. The capacity of resveratrol to obstruct several cell signaling pathways that control tumor cell invasion, metastasis, proliferation, apoptosis, inflammation, and angiogenesis may be the cause of its anti-cancer effects. Resveratrol increases chemosensitivity by reducing the function of membrane transporters including P-gp- and MDR-associated protein [23, 24]. In the chemoresistant KBv200 human oral epidermoid carcinoma cells, resveratrol increased daunorubicin accumulation in a concentration-dependent manner. In the study, researchers investigated whether resveratrol would increase the sensitivity of KBv200 cells to the chemotherapeutic medicines doxorubicin, paclitaxel, and vincristine [23]. When merged with multiple chemotherapeutic drugs, resveratrol improved the MDR phenotype of KBv200 cells by downregulating P-gp and inducing cell death [23, 24]. Numerous human cancer cell lines that have developed a resistance to multiple drugs, such as those of the colon (HT-29), abdomen (EPG85-257), and pancreas (EPG85-257), are susceptible to compounds derived from methanol extracts of *Euphorbia* spp (EPP85-181) [25]. These compounds include steroids, a diterpene, a diterpenic lactone, a polycyclic diterpene, a triterpene, and a few more related compounds. In order to determine the relative cytotoxicity of each drug, the author performed cell proliferation tests to determine their IC50 values. In contrast to their drug-resistant forebears, most cancer sublines generated as a result of drug-resistant parents showed improved sensitivity to test chemicals. The latilagascenes C and D, as well as the diterpenic lactones 3b-acetoxy-helioscopinolide B and helioscopinolide E, have been shown to have solid anticancer effects in *in vitro* experiments using the gastric carcinoma-derived, drug-resistant subline EPG85-257RDB. Against the MDR variant HT29RNOV, the macrocyclic lathyrane diterpene jolkinol B is quite effective [25].

4.4 Qualea Species and Their Medical Applications

There are more than two hundred tree and shrub species in the Vochysiaceae family [26, 27], which consists of eight different genera. Brazilian flora has several species from six South American genera. The Central Brazilian Plateau and the Guyana–Amazonian area serve as the dispersion hubs. These hubs seem to be the starting points for their expansion into neighboring neotropical and paleotropical regions [28–30].

Callisthene, Qualea, Ruizteranea, Salvertia, and Vochysia make up the Vochysiaceae [31, 32], whereas Erisma and Erismadelphus make up the Erismeae. Erismadelphus is endemic to Africa's tropics. Korupodendron is a brand-new genus consisting of a single species from western Africa [27]. It is possible to tell each of these genera apart just by looking at their flowers.

Although members of the Qualea family may be found from Mexico to Brazil's southernmost point across tropical America, the Cerrado is where they flourish. This plant is also known by the common names cassava and quaruba [33]. There are many multiple kinds of quince (Q.), but some of the most common are *Q. calantha*, *Q. cordata Spreng.*, *Q. dichotoma* (Mart.) Warm., *Q. glauca* Warm., *Q. impexa*, *Q. grandiflora* Mart., *Q. ingens* Warm. (known as arraya'n in Colombia), and *Q. multiflora* Mart. Proton pump inhibitors are effective in the leaves of this genus of plants, while topical antiseptics have been found to be efficacious in the shells and tea powder of the same species (as proved by Potts and Potts [34]). In addition, *Q grandiflora's* inner sheets and shells may be used to clean lesions, relieve external irritation, and stop diarrhea [34].

Antimicrobial and antiulcer properties of *Q. grandiflora* have been shown in studies [35, 36]. A further study found that *Q. grandiflora* had analgesic and anticonvulsant activity in the central nervous system, supporting the previous findings [37]. A decoction made from the leaves of the plant Qualea spp. has been suggested as a treatment for amebiasis, bloody diarrhea, gastritis, intestinal pain, and ulcers by Grandi *et al.* Researchers have found that *Qualea grandiflora* and *Q. multiflora* extracts are cytotoxic to tumor cells [38–41]. These extracts include ellagic acid derivatives.

4.5 Antitumor Activity of Qualea Grandiflora and Qualea Multiflora

The Brazilian Cerrado is where two types of Quince used in complementary and alternative medicine: *Q. multiflora* Mart. and *Q. grandiflora* Mart.

For instance, Carli *et al.* [40] and Quilles *et al.* [41] studied the effects of these herbs on the Ehrlich (MDR) and LM3 breast cancer cell lines in our lab. The MTT assay was used to examine the cytotoxic effects of the hexane extract, terpenoid fraction, b-sitosterol, and the terpenoid fraction from the *Q. multiflora* chloroform extract on tumor cells. Researcher also looked at how these natural substances affected immune cells, given the importance of the immune system in halting tumor development.

A terpenoid fraction of a *Q. multiflora* chloroform extract was found to be cytotoxic towards the LM3 cell line (macrophages and lymphocytes). It was revealed that Ehrlich cells were more sensitive to the b-sitosterol (obtained from the bark) and the hexane extract of *Q. grandiflora*, whereas the terpenoid fraction and macrophages were less impacted. The *Q. multiflora* terpenoid fraction's very high selective toxicity against LM3 cells was demonstrated by the treatment's nearly 100% effect on macrophage and lymphocyte vitality and 0% effect on LM3 tumor cell viability.

The gold standard medication taxol served as a comparison. Despite taxol's extensive use in cancer treatment, *in vitro* tests revealed that it did not significantly beat the *Q. grandiflora* hexane extract in terms of cytotoxicity against LM3 cells. Not only did taxol significantly reduce macrophage viability, but at higher doses, it was more hazardous to macrophages than LM3 cells. When compared to taxol, the findings from *Q. multiflora* show that its terpenoid component is more selectively cytotoxic.

4.6 Conclusion

To effectively attack multi-drug-resistant (MDR) cancer cells, new therapies must be developed, since tumors may develop resistance to most chemotherapeutic medicines. More effective treatment options may be developed if the processes by which cancer cells become resistant to chemotherapeutic drugs are better understood.

With this information and the findings reported in this chapter, the author conclude that the elements of various plants hold promise as anticancer medicines against MDR cells. Research should focus on the species of Qualea that have shown specific action against breast carcinoma cells. These results emphasize the need to further investigate promising species and the vast potential of the plant variety in the hunt for treatments for diseases like cancer. Based on these encouraging findings, more research is needed to discover alternative cancer therapy methods.

References

1. Turk, D., Hall, M.D., Chu, B.F., Ludwig, J.A., Fales, H.M., Gottesman, M.M. *et al.*, Identification of compounds selectively killing multi-drug-resistant cancer cells. *Cancer Res.*, 69, 8293e301, 2009.
2. Szakacs, G., Paterson, J.K., Ludwig, J.A., Genthe, C.B., Gottesman, M.M., Targeting multi-drug resistance in cancer. *Nature*, 5, 219e34, 2006.
3. Danial, N. and Korsmeyer, S.J., Cell death: Critical control points. *Cell*, 116, 205e19, 2004.
4. Youle, R.J. and Strasser, A., The BCL-2 protein family: Opposing activities that mediate cell death. *Nat. Rev. Mol. Cell Biol.*, 9, 47e59, 2008.
5. Lai, F., Chen, J., Farrelly, C., Margaret, L., Zhang, X., Hersey, P., Evidence for upregulation of Bim and the splicing factor SRp55 in melanoma cells from patients treated with selective BRAF inhibitors. *Melanoma Res.*, 22, 244e51, 2012.
6. Letai, A., Puma strikes Bax. *J. Cell Biol.*, 185, 189e91, 2009.
7. Becattini, B., Kitada, S., Leone, M., Monosov, E., Chandler, S., Zhai, D. *et al.*, Rational design and real time, in-cell detection of the proapoptotic activity of a novel compound targeting Bcl-X(L). *Chem. Biol.*, 11, 389e95, 2004.
8. Miller, K.D., Sweeney, C.J., Sledge Jr., G.W., Can tumor angiogenesis be inhibited without resistance? *Exp. Suppl.*, 2, 95e112, 2005.
9. Kerbe, R.S., Yu, J., Tran, J., Man, S., Viloria-Petit, A., Klement, G. *et al.*, Possible mechanisms of acquired resistance to anti-angiogenic drugs: Implications for the use of combination therapy approaches. *Cancer Metastasis Rev.*, 20, 79e86, 2001.
10. Casanovas, O., Hicklin, D.J., Bergers, G., Hanahan, D., Drug resistance by evasion of antiangiogenic targeting of VEGF signaling in late-stage pancreatic islet tumors. *Cancer Cell*, 8, 299e309, 2005.

11. Blouw, B., Song, H., Tihan, T., Bosze, J., Ferrara, N., Gerber, H. *et al.*, The hypoxic response of tumors is dependent on their microenvironment. *Cancer Cell*, 4, 133e46, 2003.
12. Carmeliet, P., Angiogenesis in life, disease and medicine. *Nature*, 438, 932e6, 2005.
13. Bergers, G. and Hanahan, D., Modes of resistance to anti-angiogenic therapy. *Nat. Rev. Cancer*, 8, 592e603, 2008.
14. Imamura, K., Okano, M., Fukamiya, N., Tagahara, K., Lee, K., Three new cytotoxic quassinoids from Brucea antidysenterica. *J. Nat. Prod.*, 56, 2091e7, 1993.
15. Fernandes, J., Castilho, R.O., Costa, M.R., WagnerSouza, K., Kaplan, M.A.C., Gattass, C.R., Pentacyclic triterpenes from Chrysobalanaceae species: Cytotoxicity on multi-drug resistant and sensitive leukemia cell lines. *Cancer Lett.*, 190, 165e9, 2003.
16. Murakami, C., Fukamya, N., Tamura, S., Okano, M., Bostow, K.F., Tokuda, H. *et al.*, Multi-drug-resistant cancer cell susceptibility to cytotoxic quassinoids and cancer chemopreventive effects os quassinoids and canthin alkaloids. *Bioorg. Med. Chem.*, 12, 4963e8, 2004.
17. Almeida, M.M.B., Arriaga, A.M.C., Santos, A.K.L., Lemos, T.L.G., Filho, R.B., Vieira, I.J.C., Occurrence and biological activity of quassinoids in the last decade. *Quim. Nova*, 30, 935e51, 2007.
18. Limtrakul, P., Siwanon, S., Yodkeereea, S., Duangrat, C., Effect of Stemona curtisii root extract on P-glycoprotein and MRP-1 functionin multi-drug-resistant cancer cells. *Phytomed*, 14, 381e9, 2007.
19. Yang, L., Wei, D.-D., Chen, Z., Wang, J.-S., Kong, L.-Y., Reversal of multi-drug resistance in human breast cancer cells by Curcuma wenyujin and Chrysanthemum indicum. *Phytomed*, 18, 710e8, 2011.
20. Suttana, W., Mankhetkorn, S., Poompimon, W., Palagani, A., Zhokhov, S., Gerlo, S. *et al.*, Differential chemosensitization of P-glycoprotein over-expressing K562/Adr cells by withaferin A and Siamois polyphenols. *Mol. Cancer*, 3, 9e99, 2010.
21. Zand, H., Chemopreventive and chemosensitization potential of flavonoids in acute lymphoblastic leukemia. *J. Pediatr. Biochem.*, 2, 15e21, 2012.
22. Chung, S.Y., Sung, M.K., Kim, N.H., Jang, J.O., Go, E.J., Lee, H.J., Inhibition of P-glycoprotein by natural products in human breast cancer cells. *Arch. Pharm. Res.*, 28, 823e8, 2005.
23. Quan, F., Pan, C.E., Zhang, S.Q., Yan, L.Y., Yu, L., Reversal effect of resveratrol on multi-drug resistance in KBv200 cell line. *Biomed. Pharmacother.*, 62, 622e9, 2008.
24. Gupta, S.C., Kannappan, R., Reuter, S., Kim, J.H., Aggarwal, B.B., Chemosensitization of tumors by resveratrol. *Ann. N. Y. Acad. Sci.*, 12, 150e60, 2011.

25. Lage, H., Duarte, N., Coburger, C., Hilgeroth, A., Ferreira, M.J.U., Antitumor activity of terpenoids against classical and atypical multi-drug resistant cancer cells. *Phytomed*, 17, 441e8, 2010.
26. Heywood, V., *Flowering plants of the world*, Croom Helm, London, 1985.
27. Litt, A. and Cheek, M., Korupodendron songweanum, a new genus and species of Vochysiaceae from West Central Africa. *Brittonia*, 54, 13e7, 2002.
28. Barroso, G.M., Peixoto, A.L., Ichaso, C.L.F., Costa, C.G., Guimaraes, E.F., Lima, H.C., *Sistemática de Angiospermas do Brasil*, Academic Press, Vicosa, 1984.
29. Kawasaki, M.L., Systematics of erisma (Vochysiaceae). *Mem. New York Bot. Gard.*, 81, 1e40, 1998.
30. Litt, A., *Floral morphology and phylogeny of Vochysiaceae.* PhD Thesis, University of New York, New York, City, 1999.
31. Stafleu, F.A., A monography of the Vochysiaceae. I. Salvertia and Vochysia. *Mededelingen van het Botanich Museum en Herbarium van Rijksuniversiteit te Utrecht*, 95, 397e540, 1948.
32. Marcano-Berti, L., Ruizterania. *Pittieria*, 2, 6e27, 1969.
33. Correa, M.P., *Dicionario das plantas u teis do Brasil e das exoticas cultivadas*, Ministerio da Agricultura, Rio de Janeiro, 1974.
34. Almeida, S.P., Proenca, C.E.B., Sano, S.M., Ribeiro, J.F., *Cerrado: Especies vegetais uteis*, EMBRAPA, Brasılia, 1998.
35. Hiruma-lima, C.A., Santos, L.C., Kushima, H., Pellizzon, C.H., Silveira, G.G., Vasconcelos, P.C. *et al.*, Qualea grandiflora, a Brazilian "Cerrado" medicinal plant presents an important antiulcer activity. *J. Ethopharmacol.*, 104, 207e14, 2006.
36. Costa, E.S., Hiruma-Lima, C.A., Lima, E.O., Sucupira, G.C., Bertolin, A.O., Lolis, S.F. *et al.*, Antimicrobial activity of some medicinal plants of the Cerrado. *Braz. Phytother. Res.*, 22, 705e7, 2008.
37. Gaspi, F.O., Foglio, M.A., Carvalho, J.E., Moreno, R.A., Pharmacological activities investigation of crude extracts and fractions from Qualea grandiflora Mart. *J. Ethopharmacol.*, 107, 19e24, 2006.
38. Grandi, T.S.M., Trindade, J.A., Pinto, M.J.F., Ferreira, L.L., Catella, A.C., Plantas Medicinais de Minas Gerais, Brasil. *Acta Bot. Bras.*, 3, 185e224, 1986.
39. Nasser, A.L.M., Carli, C.B.A., Rodrigues, C.M., Maia, D.C.G., Carlos, I.Z., Eberlin, M.N. *et al.*, Identification of ellagic acid derivatives in methanolic extracts from Qualea species. *Z. Naturforsch.*, 63c, 794e80, 2008.
40. Carli, C.B.A., Quilles, M.B., Vilegas, W., Carlos, I.Z., *Efeito dos componentes obtidos de Qualea multiflora sobre modelo tumoral mamario murino e sua influencia no sistema imunologico*, PhD Thesis, UNESP, Araraquara, 2012.
41. Quilles, M.B., Carli, C.B.A., Vilegas, W., Carlos, I.Z., *Qualea grandiflora e sua interface com o sistema imunologico em modelo experimental de adenocarcinoma murino*, PhD Thesis, UNESP, Araraquara, 2012.

5

Understanding of Autophagy to Combat MDR During Anticancer Therapy

Rishabha Malviya*, Arun Kumar Singh and Deepika Yadav

Abstract

Multi-drug resistance is a common consequence of prolonged treatment, leading to refractory cancer and tumor recurrence (MDR). This is why it is crucial to work for a world free of MDR. Treatment for both sensitive and multi-drug-resistant cancers triggers autophagy, the body's natural self-degradation mechanism. Despite its potential for killing multi-drug-resistant cancer cells (MDR C cells) when apoptotic pathways are dormant, autophagy also contributes to the growth of MDR tumors and shields C cells from chemotherapeutics. Anticancer medicines may reverse multi-drug resistance by inducing autophagy, which then triggers apoptotic signaling pathways in MDR cells. Consequently, studies into the control of autophagy as a means of combating MDR have gained prominence in recent years. In this article, the author summarize what is currently known about the function of autophagy in multi-drug-resistant tumors.

Keywords: Autophagy, drug resistance, cell death, anticancer therapy, phagophore assembly

5.1 Introduction

In order to maintain the metabolic balance, continual formation and breakdown are required for all biological processes. Proteins with a short half-life are degraded by the ubiquitin-proteasome route, whereas longer-lived macromolecular complexes and organelles are broken down via the autophagosome system [1, 2]. Recent studies reveal that abnormalities in autophagy may have significant repercussions for proper embryonic differentiation, adding to the growing body of evidence demonstrating the

**Corresponding author*: rishabhamalviya19@gmail.com

Rishabha Malviya, Arun Kumar Singh and Deepika Yadav. Multi-Drug Resistance in Cancer: Mechanism and Treatment Strategies, (87–104) © 2023 Scrivener Publishing LLC

importance of autophagy in maintaining cellular homeostasis. Several diseases, including Alzheimer's, cancer, and bacterial infections, have been associated with autophagy [3, 4]. Autophagy, the selective breakdown and recycling of cytoplasmic components, helps cells keep their energy levels stable. Microautophagy, MPIC, and ATPase autophagy are the main types of autophagy [5]. Macroautophagy and autophagy have become more interchangeable in popular use as more is learnt about both processes.

First, a specialized membrane called a phagophore has to form. The phagophore, storage for autophagy proteins, is often shown in diagrams as a tube. At maturity, when proteins with lengthy half-lives or dysfunctional organelles are present, this lipid bilayer generates a double membrane. Autolysosomes are responsible for degrading and recycling cellular components such as proteins, lipids, and nucleotides [4, 6] to keep the cell alive and functioning. An increase in autophagy has been linked to both chemotherapy and sickness progression. However, not all cancer cells benefit from chemotherapy since autophagy has been linked to cancer drug resistance and refractoriness [7].

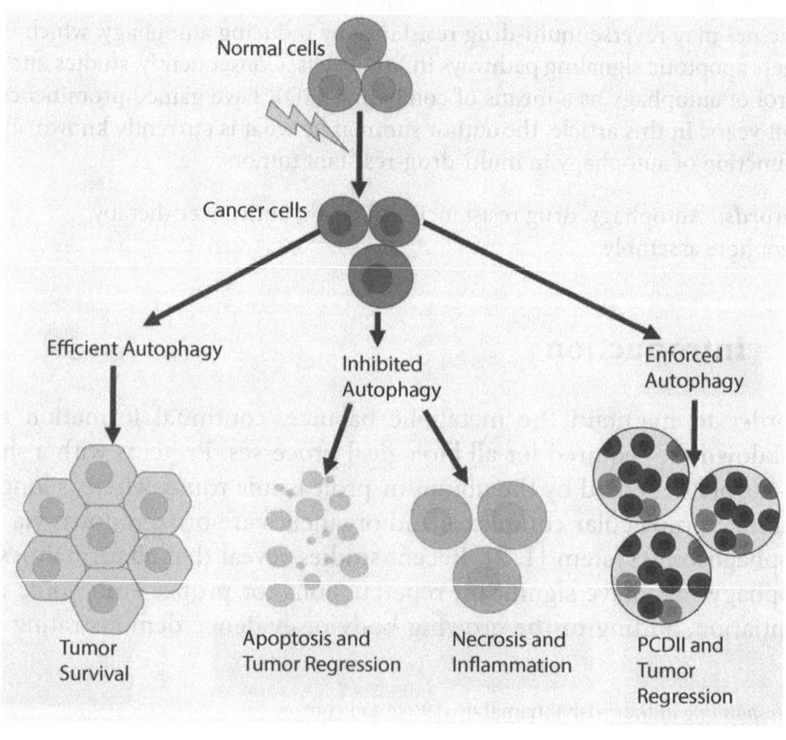

Figure 5.1 Schematic representation of cancerous autophagy and the development of drug resistance.

Multi-drug resistance (MDR) is another undesirable outcome of chemotherapy, in which cells become resistant to many chemotherapeutic agents despite fundamental variations in their structure and function [8]. Multi-drug resistance contributes to the failure of "chemotherapy" and the resulting increase in cancer mortality. There is evidence from recent mechanistic investigations [9] linking autophagy pathways to the development of MDR. However, our understanding of the processes involved in autophagy hijacking, which has been examined as a viable weapon in the fight against cancer, is lacking. This is particularly true in the case of multi-drug-resistant cancer cells. Cancerous autophagy and the development of drug resistance are successfully depicted in Figure 5.1.

5.2 Mechanisms of Autophagy

Autophagy is a process that occurs often in almost all cells. There are around 30 genes (Atgs) that have been singled out as crucial for autophagy in yeast, and there have been reports of additional genetic homologs in mammals [10]. Cells rely on Atgs to adapt to environmental stresses such as hypoxia, heat stress, and reactive oxygen species (ROS) production. Phagophore development, autophagosome maturation, and lysosome fusion are the first steps in autophagy [11, 12]. There is a quick overview of some of the primary routes that control autophagy.

5.2.1 Phagophore Assembly

The autophagosome's membrane core first expands to a particular size throughout development. Autophagosome assembly requires the adaptor protein Atg13, the serine/threonine-protein kinase ULK1, and the tight junction kinase (FAK) family kinase-interacting peptide 200 [13, 14]. (FIP200). The autophagosomal membrane contains much more phosphatidylinositol 3-phosphate (PI3P) than other cell membranes [15]. Class III PtdIns3K complexes control the formation of autophagosomes [16], a process that requires PtdIns(3)P-rich membranes. In particular, a complex composed of Vps34, Vps15, Beclin1, and Atg14 is important in vacuolar protein sorting. Beclin1 is necessary for the proper functioning of the Ambra1-DLC1 (ubiquitin-like modifier 1) protein secreted by the dynein motor complex [17]. Beclin1 requires ULK1 in order to function normally. The autophagosome's membranes have been shown to have descended from the ER and the Golgi [18]. The phagophore served as a junction for mitochondrial and ER communication [19]. The plasma membrane and endosomes are necessary for the development of autophagosomes [20].

5.2.2 Autophagosome Formation and Maturation

The Atg12 conjugation system generates double-membrane autophagosomes for waste transport and digestion, as well as regulating autophagy initiation and phagophore synthesis. Atg12 is covalently conjugated to Atg5 in this system through an E1-like enzyme, Atg7, and an E2-like enzyme, Atg10 [21]. The Atg12–Atg5–Atg16 (L1) complex quickly binds autophagosome membranes [22], despite being formed late in autophagosome formation. Particularly, it interacts with a protein called MAP1LC3, which improves microtubule assembly. The first stage of the LC3 pathway involves phosphatidylethanolamine, during which LC3 binds to the (PE). Atg4 lip oxidizes LC3, creating LC3-I, which readily connects to PE [23]. This results in significant time savings. Both the E1-like enzyme Atg7 and the E2-like enzyme Atg3 are necessary for PE conjugation to the C-terminal glycine of LC3-I [24].

5.2.3 Autolysosome Degradation

The autolysosome, formed when an autophagosome fuse with a lysosome, is responsible for degradation by disassembling the degradation target into its constituent parts. Membrane-bound structures called autophagosomes contain LC3 protein conjugates (PE). Lysosomal proteases cleave LC3-PE on the autophagosome's inner membrane to facilitate the recycling of amino acids, fatty acids, and nucleotides [25], whereas Atg4 cleaves and recycles the outer membrane.

5.2.4 Core Regulator of Autophagy

Protein kinase mTOR controls autophagy, which promotes cell growth and survival. The sensory receptor mTOR may be activated by a wide variety of stimuli, including drugs, low oxygen levels, UV radiation, and fluctuations in the intracellular concentration of amino acids, glucose, and other chemicals. When intracellular resources are plentiful, activating the mammalian target of rapamycin (mTOR) may protect cells against proteolysis and autophagy [26]. Dephosphorylation of ULK1 is mediated via phosphorylation of Atg13 and RB1-inducible coiled-coil (1RB1CC1/FIP200), shielding the organism from the deleterious effects of hunger.

Type III phosphatidylinositol 3-kinase (PIK3C3/VPS34) has been connected *in vitro* and *in vivo* to the inactivation of the mammalian target of rapamycin complex 1 (mTORC1) [27]. The PIK3C3/VPS34 inhibitor SAR405 adds to the growing body of evidence demonstrating the importance of mTOR kinase control in autophagy [28]. Acting via mTOR, PIK3C3 controls lysosomal repopulation and autolysosomal tubule sorting directly [29].

5.3 Mechanisms of MDR

Mechanisms for preventing the activation of apoptotic signaling pathways include lowering drug uptake by influx hauliers, such as solute carriers [30], lowering drug exudation by membrane proteins with Kinase cassette (ABC) isoforms acting as the primary transporters [31], and so on. Figure 5.2 shows the mechanism of MDR.

Based on sequence and structural similarities, ABC transporters may be divided into seven subfamilies, called ABC-A through ABC-G [9]. P-glycoprotein (P-gp/ABCB1), multi-drug-resistant protein 1 (MRP1/ABCC1) [32–35], breast cancer-resistant protein (BCRP/ABCG2/MXR/ABCP) [36–38], and multi-drug-resistant protein 10 (ABCC10/MRP7) [39, 40] are all examples of transporters that are often seen pushing chemosensitive tumors toward MDR [41]. Although several members of the ABC

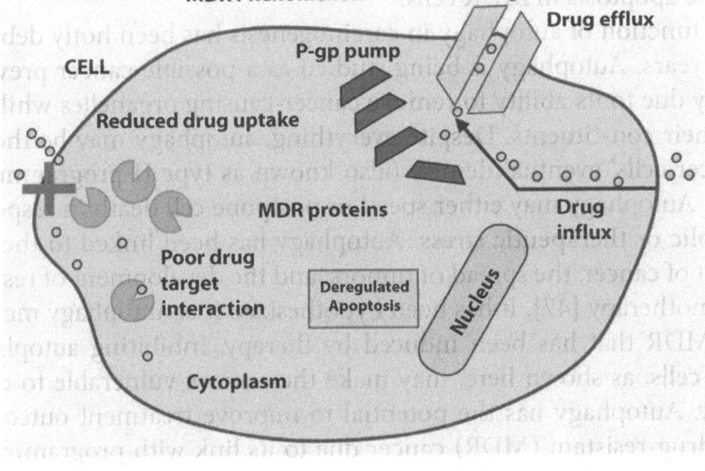

Figure 5.2 Schematic representation of the mechanism of MDR.

transporter family have been identified in other organisms, only ABCB1 has been identified in humans. Part chemotherapeutic medicines lose some of their effectiveness when ABCB1 is overexpressed. Many studies have shown that ABCC1 is associated with cancer cell resistance to mitoxantrone, saquinavir, epipodophyllotoxins, and anthracyclines [42–45]. ABCG2 transporter expression is much greater in ovarian, breast, colon, stomach, and small-cell lung tumors than in other malignancies [31]. ABC transporter activity is highly associated with the occurrence of MDR. The development of medicines to block or shut down ABC transporters has been linked to an increase in the efficacy of anticancer medications [46].

5.4 Correlation Between Autophagy and Multi-Drug Resistance

Cancer might theoretically be cured by chemotherapy since it causes cancer cells to destroy themselves. The failure to properly undergo apoptosis has been connected to the evolution of drug resistance, as shown by a number of studies. Given that MDR cancer cells are resistant to several standard anticancer treatments, medications must be developed that can selectively target and kill these cells. However, developing a treatment to inhibit apoptosis takes far more time and energy. Drug resistance is a major problem in public health, and it is generally the consequence of chronic exposure to a novel chemical. It has been theorized by researchers that autophagy may promote apoptosis in MDR cells.

The function of autophagy in carcinogenesis has been hotly debated in recent years. Autophagy is being studied as a possible cancer prevention strategy due to its ability to remove cancer-causing organelles while recycling their constituents. Despite everything, autophagy may be the cause of cancer cells' eventual demise (also known as type II programmed cell death). Autophagy may either speed or postpone cell death in response to metabolic or therapeutic stress. Autophagy has been linked to the development of cancer, the spread of tumors, and the development of resistance to chemotherapy [47]. It has been hypothesized that autophagy may overcome MDR that has been induced by therapy. Inhibiting autophagy in cancer cells, as shown here, may make them more vulnerable to chemotherapy. Autophagy has the potential to improve treatment outcomes in multi-drug-resistant (MDR) cancer due to its link with programmed cell death (apoptosis); nevertheless, its significance in MDR must be extensively investigated.

5.5 The Cytoprotective Effect of Autophagy in the Regulation of Multi-Drug Resistance

Researchers have shown that concentrating on ABC transporters may help in the development of anti-MDR medications. However, studies on people using currently available ABC transporter modulators have not shown promising results. And MDR is a complex personality quirk. The putative association between autophagy and MDR has been the subject of many clinical data analyses. New evidence linking autophagy to cancer development, metastasis, and medication resistance was discovered using tumor samples from persons who had survived colorectal cancer for at least 5 years [48]. The expression of ABCB1 is associated favorably with that of LC3, Beclin1, and Rictor, but adversely with Raptor.

5.6 Increased Autophagy Facilitates Multi-Drug Resistance

Multiple pieces of evidence point to the co-occurrence of autophagy and MDR. The fast emergence of One's prognosis tends to worsen when autophagy is present, and it has been related to MDR and other negative outcomes. Despite this, Yang *et al*'s suggest that autophagy in leukemia cells may be regulated, hence lowering their multi-drug resistance [49]. Adriamycin and vincristine stimulate the production of S100A8, a protein required for the formation of the Beclin1-Class III phosphatidylinositol 3-kinase (PI3KC3) complex [49, 50]. It has been hypothesized that proteins like high-mobility group box 1 (HMGB1) govern drug resistance in cancer, and this connection has been made between autophagy and the therapeutic benefits of chemotherapy (MDR). The binding of cytoplasmic HMGB1 to its receptor stimulates the development of a beclin1-PI3KC3 complex, which in turn triggers the MAPK/ERK signaling cascade [51]. According to the research of Fan *et al.*, hepatocellular carcinoma cells may become more resistant to treatment if autophagy is induced in them [52].

MiRNAs have been discovered to target Atgs in MDR cancer cells, where they play a crucial role. Xu *et al.* have shown that miR-199a-5p downregulation may activate autophagy, which in turn provides resistance to cisplatin [53]. Targeting Atg5 with MiR-181a increases cisplatin's cytotoxicity *in vitro* and *in vivo* in cisplatin-selective MDR SGC7901/CDDP cells [54].

Autophagy in cancer cells has been related to the development of resistance to chemotherapeutic medications such paclitaxel [55], tamoxifen [56], epirubicin [57], and trastuzumab [58]. As shown by Sun *et al.*, epirubicin promoted autophagy in both parental MCF-7 cells and epirubicin-resistant MCF-7er cells [57]. Epirubicin causes apoptosis in MCF-7er cells, while autophagy provides temporary protection [57]. The chemotherapy medicines epirubicin (ER), paclitaxel (TAX), and vinorelbine (VNR) were tested on two cell lines that overexpress ABCB1 by Sun *et al.* [59]. In particular, MCF-7er and SK-BR-3er strains, are resistant to epirubicin. Scientists found that the chemotherapy drugs paclitaxel and vinorelbine activated autophagy, which protected MDR cells from cell death [59]. Although autophagy may not have a direct effect on ABCB1 expression, it unquestionably facilitates the development of multi-drug resistance.

Table 5.1 Recent studies on the pro-survival role of autophagy in multi-drug-resistant (MDR) cancer [66].

Intervention for tumor treatment	Cell line	Method to study autophagy
miR-23b-3p	Vincristine-resistant SGC7901	CQ, siRNAs (Atg12, HMGB2)
5-FU	Drug-resistant esophageal cancer cells	3-MA, siRNAs (Beclin1, Atg7)
Epirubicin	Epirubicin-resistant MDA-MB-231	CQ
Ursolic acid	*PTEN*-deficient PC3	3-MA, siRNAs (Atg5, Beclin1)
PI-103	Cisplatin-resistant ovarian cancer cells	siRNAs (Beclin1, LC3), Baf A1
PP2	Ras-NIH3T3/Mdr	3-MA
Suberoylanilide hydroxamic acid	Imatinib-resistant CML cells	CQ
B-raf inhibitors	B-Raf inhibitor-resistant melanoma cells	HCQ
Cisplatin	Cisplatin-resistant A549/DDP	3-MA
Docetaxel	Adriamycin-resistant MCF-7	CQ
Doxorubicin	Adriamycin-resistant MCF-7	CQ
Vincristine	VCR-resistant ovarian carcinoma SKVCR	3-MA, CQ

5.7 Autophagy Inhibition Improves Chemotherapy in MDR Cancers

In light of growing evidence that MDR triggers autophagy, many innovative therapeutic approaches have been proposed (Table 5.1). Genetic suppression of Atgs including Beclin1, Atg5, Atg7, and Atg12 has been shown to reduce autophagy and increase drug responsiveness in multi-drug-resistant (MDR) cells [60–62]. In the cancer cell line SGC7901/VCR, overexpression of Atg12 and high-mobility group box 2 leads to resistance to the chemotherapeutic drug vincristine and an increase in autophagy (HMGB2). *In vitro* and *in vivo* research has revealed that overexpressing miR-23b-3p may restore chemosensitivity in MDR cells [63]. This miRNA controls the levels of Atg12 and HMGB2 in particular. By inhibiting autophagy, chemotherapeutics may be more effective against SGC7901/VCR cells. This may be done with compounds like chloroquine (CQ) [63] or herceptin-like mucin-like protein 2 (HMGB2) and Atg12 small interfering RNAs (siRNAs). When it comes to vincristine-induced multi-drug resistance, this study provides the first definitive evidence that autophagy is to blame. Some MDR cell types use a self-preservation mechanism called autophagy [64] when they are exposed to chemotherapeutic therapies like 5-fluorouracil and cisplatin, and once the medications are withdrawn, the cells rapidly revert to normal [64]. When compared to their parental lines, anthracycline-resistant MDA-MB-231-R8 and SUM159PT-R75 lines

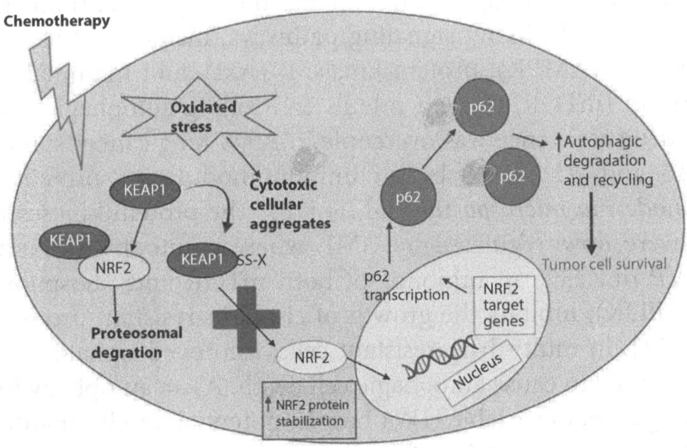

Figure 5.3 Representation of mechanism of action of autophagy inhibition improves chemotherapy in MDR cancers.

have a greater basal autophagic flux. Downregulation of Atg5 and Atg7, or pharmacological inhibition of autophagy with CQ or hydroxychloroquine (HCQ), reduces the lifespan of epirubicin-sensitive and epirubicin-resistant triple-negative breast cancer cells, respectively [65]. This study supports the theory that autophagy is used by MDR cells as a defense mechanism against anthracycline. The mechanism of action of autophagy is depicted in Figure 5.3.

5.8 Overcoming MDR With Autophagic Cell Death

This research demonstrates that autophagy facilitates autophagic cell killing in apoptosis-resistant MDR cells. Strong autophagy has been the focus of many studies because of its potential to eliminate multi-drug-resistant cancer cells. Suberoylanilide hydroxamic acid (SAHA), a histone deacetylase inhibitor that was identified very recently, effectively suppresses tumor growth [66, 67]. Induction of autophagic cell death by SAHA in tamoxifen-resistant MCF-7 breast cancer cells. The proliferation of apoptosis-resistant colon cancer cells is inhibited by two lipophilic tanshinones, cryptotanshinone, and dihydrotanshinone [68]. Vocamine [62], a bisindolic alkaloid, has the potential to trigger autophagy, which may then be used to destroy multi-drug-resistant tumor cells. Lipid nanoparticles with edelfosine have the potential to destroy the edelfosine-resistant leukemia cell line K562 [69]. These findings suggest that when apoptosis fails to eliminate MDR cells, autophagic cell death might be boosted as an additional cell death strategy.

Although autophagy may be able to kill MDR-CRCs, which are resistant to many chemotherapeutic treatments, they remain a promising target for cancer research. Many signaling pathways, including AMP-activated protein kinase (AMPK), protein kinase B (Akt), and mammalian target of rapamycin (mTOR), have a role in controlling autophagic cell death. Multiple drug resistance was overcome in A549 lung cancer sub-cell lines A549/D16 and A549/V16 by an immunomodulatory protein derived from *Ganoderma microsporum* (GMI) [70]. The protein kinases Akt and p70S6K were downregulated by GMI, whereas autophagy was upregulated. NVP-BEZ235, an inhibitor of both mTOR and phosphoinositide 3-kinase (PI3K), inhibits the growth of cisplatin-resistant urothelial cancer cells [71]. In multi-drug-resistant cells, improved signaling pathways may be required to cause autophagic cell death. As an autophagy inhibitor, human single-chain variable HW1 has the potential for eliminating tumor cells that have become resistant to a tumor necrosis factor-like apoptosis-inducing ligand (TRAIL). For HW1 to trigger autophagic cell death, the c-Jun NH2-terminal kinase pathway must be activated [72].

5.9 Autophagy Kills Apoptosis-Deficient MDR Cancer Cells

However, in multi-drug-resistant (MDR) cells, which are unable to carry out programmed cell death, the adaptive response of autophagy may confer improved resistance to chemotherapeutics. Autophagy may act as a scavenger in signaling pathways generally regulated by apoptosis, allowing MDR tumors easier access to apoptosis. Autophagy is induced in etoposide-resistant, ABCB1-overexpressed A549 cells by the novel furanocoumarin feronellin A, which was discovered in *Feroniella lucida*. The apoptosis triggered by ferroinellin A was considerably mitigated by the application of beclin1 siRNA. Combining Feroniellin A-induced cell death with the autophagy stimulant rapamycin [73] may be more successful. The autophagy-inducing effects of metformin may make TRAIL-resistant lung cancer cells more susceptible to the apoptosis-inducing effects of TRAIL. Benefits include increased autophagic flux and decreased expression of the cellular FADD-like IL-1-converting enzyme (c-FLIP) when metformin is used.

5.10 Autophagy Promotes Chemosensitivity

When multi-drug-resistant cancer cells grow reliant on autophagy for survival, this may reduce the efficacy of treatments intended to overcome drug resistance. Recent evidence, however, suggests that autophagy induced by certain drugs may be all that is needed to overcome MDR (Figure 5.4). *In vitro* studies using underivatized fullerene C60 (nano-C60) nanocrystals have shown encouraging results in the battle against several neoplasms. Stress from nano-oxidative C60 and maybe autophagy might be amplified by photoactivation [74, 75]. Nano-sized carbon nanotubes (nano-C60) induced autophagy, which led to the death of drug-resistant MCF-7 cancer cells. Inhibiting autophagy with the reactive oxygen species (ROS) scavenger N-acetyl-l-cysteine may mitigate the nano-chemosensitizing effects of C60. The key to this tactic is Atg5, since suppressing it (Atg5 siRNA/) or knocking it out (Atg5/) protects cells against the chemosensitivity produced by nano-C60 [76, 77]. In addition, a nano-C60 derivative with increased activity may induce autophagy, which may sensitize doxorubicin-resistant MCF-7 cells [77]. Since cysteine stimulates autophagy *in vitro* and *in vivo* [78], it is likely that doxorubicin-resistant MCF-7/ADR cells would react to doxorubicin and doxorubicin combination therapy. Our results support the idea that autophagy may help reverse MDR, even if the underlying

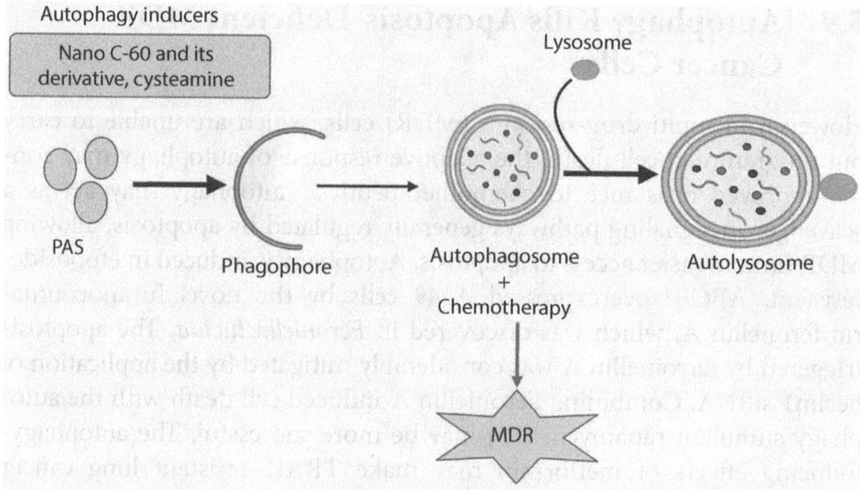

Figure 5.4 When autophagy is activated, drug-resistant cancer cells become more sensitive to therapy.

molecular pathways are still poorly understood. The sensitivity of drug-resistant cancer cells to therapy is shown in Figure 5.4.

Initiating autophagy is a new function of cysteamine, nano-C60 (underivatized fullerene C60), and its derivative. Multi-drug-resistant (MDR) cancer cells that undergo autophagy in response to these inducers may become more susceptible to chemotherapeutics.

5.11 Conclusion

Research on autophagy and its dual role in multi-drug resistance has exploded in recent years. Autophagy may either hasten cell death or improve cell survival, and this effect can vary depending on the kind of tumor and the treatment strategy. Inhibiting autophagy may render cancer cells more susceptible to chemotherapy, despite the fact that it shields them from death and boosts resistance to treatment. Studies have revealed that cytotoxic drugs are more effective when autophagy is suppressed. Combining CQ or HCQ with other cancer medicines authorized by the FDA may boost the cytotoxicity of the combination, allowing for more effective treatment of previously unresponsive tumors. Tumors that have developed resistance to standard treatments will be the target of these new drugs. When induced by autophagy inducers, autophagic cell death may be an alternative to apoptosis for eliminating MDR cells. An exciting new phase in the fight against cancers that have become resistant to standard therapy has begun. More and more evidence suggests that autophagy is not only a potent propellant but also crucial for reversing MDR and rendering apoptosis-resistant MDR cells susceptible to anticancer therapies. This provides more proof of autophagy's biological role in MDR cancer cells and opens the door to potential novel treatments for the condition. Autophagy and the eradication of multi-drug resistance are two such processes that have a limited understanding but might benefit from more study. As research into MDR has exploded over the last several years, so too has the discussion of the twin function autophagy plays in MDR. Depending on the kind of tumor and the therapy, autophagy may either speed up cancer cell death or increase their potential to survive. By decreasing protection against apoptosis and increasing resistance to chemotherapy, inhibiting autophagy may render multi-drug-resistant cancer cells more susceptible to anticancer treatments. For some time now, the combination of anti-autophagy medications with cytotoxic treatments has been thought to be the most effective. Increasing cytotoxicity and making previously drug-resistant tumors more treatable are two benefits of combining CQ or HCQ with other anticancer medications authorized by the FDA. Tumors that have developed resistance to standard treatments will be the target of these new drugs. Apoptosis is not the only way to get rid of MDR cells; autophagic cell death, induced by autophagy inducers, may occur as well. This resistance has opened a new front in the battle against cancer, which was formerly treatable. Autophagy has been shown to be a potent propellant in the fight against cancer, as well as a crucial factor in reversing MDR and rendering apoptosis-resistant MDR cells accessible to anticancer therapy. This demonstrates the importance of autophagy in MDR cancer cells biologically and provides the path for novel approaches to combating this threat. Despite the present lack of clarity on the mechanisms involved, the intriguing link between autophagy and MDR reversal provides a strong foundation for researching and, perhaps, shedding light on the systems involved.

References

1. Boya, P., Reggiori, F., Codogno, P., Emerging regulation and functions of autophagy. *Nat. Cell Biol.*, 15, 8, 713–20, 2013.
2. Deschenes-Simard, X., Lessard, F., Gaumont-Leclerc, M.F., Bardeesy, N., Ferbeyre, G., Cellular senescence and protein degradation breaking down cancer. *Cell Cycle*, 13, 12, 1840–58, 2014.
3. Levine, B. and Kroemer, G., Autophagy in the pathogenesis of disease. *Cell*, 132, 1, 27–42, 2008.
4. Sridhar, S., Botbol, Y., Macian, F., Cuervo, A.M., Autophagy and disease: Always two sides to a problem. *J. Pathol.*, 226, 2, 255–73, 2012.

5. Chiang, H.L., Terlecky, S.R., Plant, C.P., Dice, J.F., A role for a 70-kilodalton heat shock protein in lysosomal degradation of intracellular proteins. *Science*, 246, 4928, 382–5, 1989.
6. Hundeshagen, P., Hamacher-Brady, A., Eils, R., Brady, N.R., Concurrent detection of autolysosome formation and lysosomal degradation by flow cytometry in a high-content screen for inducers of autophagy. *BMC Biol.*, 9, 38, 2011.
7. Buchser, W.J., Laskow, T.C., Pavlik, P.J., Lin, H.M., Lotze, M.T., Cell-mediated autophagy promotes cancer cell survival. *Cancer Res.*, 72, 12, 2970–9, 2012.
8. Holohan, C., Van Schaeybroeck, S., Longley, D.B., Johnston, P.G., Cancer drug resistance: An evolving paradigm. *Nat. Rev. Cancer*, 13, 10, 714–26, 2013.
9. Kumar, P., Zhang, D.M., Degenhardt, K., Chen, Z.S., Autophagy and transporter-based multi-drug resistance. *Cells*, 1, 3, 558–75, 2012.
10. Klionsky, D.J., Look people, "Atg" is an abbreviation for "autophagy-related." That's it. *Autophagy*, 8, 9, 1281–2, 2012.
11. Ganley, I.G., Wong, P.M., Gammoh, N., Jiang, X.J., Distinct autophagosomal-lysosomal fusion mechanism revealed by thapsigargin-induced autophagy arrest. *Mol. Cell*, 42, 6, 731–43, 2011.
12. Suzuki, K., Kirisako, T., Kamada, Y., Mizushima, N., Noda, T., Ohsumi, Y., The pre-autophagosomal structure organized by concerted functions of APG genes is essential for autophagosome formation. *EMBO J.*, 20, 21, 5971–81, 2001.
13. Chan, E.Y.W., Kir, S., Tooze, S.A., SiRNA screening of the kinome identifies ULK1 as a multidomain modulator of autophagy. *J. Biol. Chem.*, 282, 35, 25464–74, 2007.
14. Hara, T., Takamura, A., Kishi, C., Iemura, S.I., Natsume, T., Guan, J.L. *et al.*, FIP200, a ULK-interacting protein, is required for autophagosome formation in mammalian cells. *J. Cell Biol.*, 181, 3, 497–510, 2008.
15. Obara, K., Noda, T., Niimi, K., Ohsumi, Y., Transport of phosphatidylino-sitol 3-phosphate into the vacuole via autophagic membranes in Saccharomyces cerevisiae. *Genes Cells*, 13, 6, 537–47, 2008.
16. Matsunaga, K., Saitoh, T., Tabata, K., Omori, H., Satoh, T., Kurotori, N. *et al.*, Two Beclin 1-binding proteins, Atg14L and Rubicon, reciprocally regulate autophagy at different stages. *Nat. Cell Biol.*, 11, 4, 385–96, 2009.
17. Fimia, G.M., Di Bartolomeo, S., Piacentini, M., Cecconi, F., Unleashing the Ambra1-Beclin 1 complex from dynein chains Ulk1 sets Ambra1 free to induce autophagy. *Autophagy*, 7, 1, 115–7, 2011.
18. Ge, L., Melville, D., Zhang, M., Schekman, R., The ER-Golgi intermediate compartment is a key membrane source for the LC3 lipidation step of autophagosome biogenesis. *Elife*, 2, 00947, 2013.
19. Hamasaki, M., Furuta, N., Matsuda, A., Nezu, A., Yamamoto, A., Fujita, N. *et al.*, Autophagosomes form at ER-mitochondria contact sites. *Nature*, 495, 7441, 389–93, 2013.
20. Puri, C., Renna, M., Bento, C.F., Moreau, K., Rubinsztein, D.C., Diverse autophago-some membrane sources coalesce in recycling endosomes. *Cell*, 154, 6, 1285–99, 2013.

21. Mizushima, N., Noda, T., Yoshimori, T., Tanaka, Y., Ishii, T., George, M.D. *et al.*, A protein conjugation system essential for autophagy. *Nature*, 395, 6700, 395–8, 1998.
22. Fujioka, Y., Noda, N.N., Nakatogawa, H., Ohsumi, Y., Inagaki, F., Dimeric coiled-coil structure of Saccharomyces cerevisiae Atg16 and its functional significance in autophagy. *J. Biol. Chem.*, 285, 2, 1508–15, 2010.
23. Romanov, J., Walczak, M., Ibiricu, I., Schuchner, S., Ogris, E., Kraft, C. *et al.*, Mechanism and functions of membrane binding by the Atg5-Atg12/Atg16 complex during autophagosome formation. *EMBO J.*, 31, 22, 4304–17, 2012.
24. Ichimura, Y., Kirisako, T., Takao, T., Satomi, Y., Shimonishi, Y., Ishihara, N. *et al.*, A ubiquitin-like system mediates protein lipidation. *Nature*, 408, 6811, 488–92, 2000.
25. Singh, R. and Cuervo, A.M., Autophagy in the cellular energetic balance. *Cell Metab.*, 13, 5, 495–504, 2011.
26. Alers, S., Loffler, A.S., Wesselborg, S., Stork, B., Role of AMPK-mTOR-Ulk1/2 in the regulation of autophagy: Cross talk, shortcuts, and feedbacks. *Mol. Cell Biol.*, 32, 1, 2–11, 2012.
27. Yuan, H.X., Russell, R.C., Guan, K.L., Regulation of PIK3C3/VPS34 complexes by MTOR in nutrient stress-induced autophagy. *Autophagy*, 9, 12, 1983–95, 2013.
28. Pasquier, B., SAR405, a PIK3C3/Vps34 inhibitor that prevents autophagy and synergizes with MTOR inhibition in tumor cells. *Autophagy*, 11, 4, 725, 2015.
29. Yu, L., McPhee, C.K., Zheng, L.X., Mardones, G.A., Rong, Y.G., Peng, J.Y. *et al.*, Termination of autophagy and reformation of lysosomes regulated by mTOR. *Nature*, 465, 7300, 942–6, 2010.
30. Chun, S.Y., Kwon, Y.S., Nam, K.S., Kim, S., Lapatinib enhances the cytotoxic effects of doxorubicin in MCF-7 tumorspheres by inhibiting the drug efflux function of ABC transporters. *Biomed. Pharmacother.*, 72, 37–43, 2015.
31. Giacomini, K.M., Huang, S.M., Tweedie, D.J., Benet, L.Z., Brouwer, K.L.R., Chu, X.Y. *et al.*, Membrane transporters in drug development. *Nat. Rev. Drug Discovery*, 9, 3, 215–36, 2010.
32. Filomeni, G., Turella, P., Dupuis, M.L., Forini, O., Ciriolo, M.R., Cianfriglia, M. *et al.*, 6-(7-Nitro-2,1,3-benzoxadiazol-4-ylthio)hexanol, a specific glutathione S-transferase inhibitor, overcomes the multi-drug resistance (MDR)-associated protein 1-mediated MDR in small cell lung cancer. *Mol. Cancer Ther.*, 7, 2, 371–9, 2008.
33. Rodriguez-Antona, C. and Ingelman-Sundberg, M., Cytochrome P450 pharmacogenetics and cancer. *Oncogene*, 25, 11, 1679–91, 2006.
34. Wilson, C.S., Medeiros, L.J., Lai, R., Butch, A.W., McCourty, A., Kelly, K. *et al.*, DNA topoisomerase II alpha in multiple myeloma: A marker of cell proliferation and not drug resistance. *Mod. Pathol.*, 14, 9, 886–91, 2001.
35. Bedi, A., Barber, J.P., Bedi, G.C., El-Deiry, W.S., Sidransky, D., Vala, M.S. *et al.*, BCR-ABL-mediated inhibition of apoptosis with delay of G2/M transition after DNA damage: A mechanism of resistance to multiple anticancer agents. *Blood*, 86, 3, 1148–58, 1995.

36. Shoemaker, R.H., Genetic and epigenetic factors in anticancer drug resistance. *J. Natl. Cancer Inst.*, 92, 1, 4–5, 2000.
37. Li, H. and Yang, B.B., Friend or foe: The role of microRNA in chemotherapy resistance. *Acta Pharmacol. Sin.*, 34, 7, 870–9, 2013.
38. Camidge, D.R., Pao, W., Sequist, L.V., Acquired resistance to TKIs in solid tumours: Learning from lung cancer. *Nat. Rev. Clin. Oncol.*, 11, 8, 473–81, 2014.
39. Milane, L., Duan, Z.F., Amiji, M., Role of hypoxia and glycolysis in the development of multi-drug resistance in human tumor cells and the establishment of an orthotopic multi-drug resistant tumor model in nude mice using hypoxic pre-conditioning. *Cancer Cell Int.*, 11, 3, 2011.
40. Dean, M., Fojo, T., Bates, S., Tumour stem cells and drug resistance. *Nat. Rev. Cancer*, 5, 4, 275–84, 2005.
41. Kathawala, R.J., Wang, Y.J., Ashby, C.R., Jr *et al.*, Recent advances regarding the role of ABC subfamily C member 10 (ABCC10) in the efflux of antitumor drugs. *Chin. J. Cancer*, 33, 5, 223–30, 2014.
42. Morrow, C.S., Peklak-Scott, C., Bishwokarma, B., Kute, T.E., Smitherman, P.K., Townsend, A.J., Multi-drug resistance protein 1 (MRP1, ABCC1) mediates resistance to mitoxantrone via glutathione-dependent drug efflux. *Mol. Pharmacol.*, 69, 4, 1499–1505, 2006.
43. König, S.K., Herzog, M., Theile, D., Zembruski, N., Haefeli, W.E., Weiss, J., Impact of drug transporters on cellular resistance towards saquinavir and darunavir. *J. Antimicrob. Chemother.*, 65, 11, 2319–2328, 2010.
44. Anreddy, N., Gupta, P., Kathawala, R.J., Patel, A., Wurpel, J.N., Chen, Z.S., Tyrosine kinase inhibitors as reversal agents for ABC transporter mediated drug resistance. *Molecules*, 19, 9, 13848–13877, 2014.
45. Wang, Y.J., Zhang, Y.K., Kathawala, R.J., Chen, Z.S., Repositioning of tyrosine kinase inhibitors as antagonists of ATP-binding cassette transporters in anticancer drug resistance. *Cancers*, 6, 4, 1925–1952, 2014.
46. Zhang, G.N., Ashby, C.R., Zhang, Y.K., Chen, Z.S., Guo, H., The reversal of antineoplastic drug resistance in cancer cells by β-elemene. *Chin. J. Cancer*, 34, 3, 1–8, 2015.
47. Yuan, P., Cao, W., Zang, Q., Li, G., Guo, X., Fan, J., The HIF-2α-MALAT1-miR-216b axis regulates multi-drug resistance of hepatocellular carcinoma cells via modulating autophagy. *Biochem. Biophys. Res. Commun.*, 478, 3, 1067–1073, 2016.
48. Shuhua, W., Chenbo, S., Yangyang, L.I., Xiangqian, G., Shuang, H., Tangyue, L., Dong, T., Autophagy-related genes Raptor, Rictor, and Beclin1 expression and relationship with multi-drug resistance in colorectal carcinoma. *Hum. Pathol.*, 46, 11, 1752–1759, 2015.
49. Morselli, E., Galluzzi, L., Kepp, O., Vicencio, J.M., Criollo, A., Maiuri, M.C., Kroemer, G., Anti-and pro-tumor functions of autophagy. *Biochim. Biophys. Acta (BBA)-Mol. Cell Res.*, 1793, 9, 1524–1532, 2009.
50. Mathew, R. and White, E., Autophagy in tumorigenesis and energy metabolism: Friend by day, foe by night. *Curr. Opin. Genet. Dev.*, 21, 1, 113–119, 2011.
51. Rabinowitz, J.D. and White, E., Autophagy and metabolism. *Science*, 330, 6009, 1344–1348, 2010.

52. Lebovitz, C.B., Bortnik, S.B., Gorski, S.M., Here, there be dragons: Charting autophagy-related alterations in human tumorsautophagy-related alterations in human tumors. *Clin. Cancer Res.*, 18, 5, 1214–1226, 2012.
53. Yang, S., Wang, X., Contino, G., Liesa, M., Sahin, E., Ying, H., Kimmelman, A.C., Pancreatic cancers require autophagy for tumor growth. *Genes Dev.*, 25, 7, 717–729, 2011.
54. Moreau, K., Luo, S., Rubinsztein, D.C., Cytoprotective roles for autophagy. *Curr. Opin. Cell Biol.*, 22, 206–211, 2010.
55. Sandilands, E., Serrels, B., McEwan, D.G., Morton, J.P., Macagno, J.P., McLeod, K., Frame, M.C., Autophagic targeting of Src promotes cancer cell survival following reduced FAK signalling. *Nat. Cell Biol.*, 14, 1, 51–60, 2012.
56. Rubinstein, A.D., Eisenstein, M., Ber, Y., Bialik, S., Kimchi, A., The autophagy protein Atg12 associates with antiapoptotic Bcl-2 family members to promote mitochondrial apoptosis. *Mol. Cell*, 44, 5, 698–709, 2011.
57. Guo, J.Y., Chen, H.Y., Mathew, R., Fan, J., Strohecker, A.M., Karsli-Uzunbas, G., White, E., Activated Ras requires autophagy to maintain oxidative metabolism and tumorigenesis. *Genes Dev.*, 25, 5, 460–470, 2011.
58. Kang, R., Loux, T., Tang, D., Schapiro, N.E., Vernon, P., Livesey, K.M., Zeh III, H.J., The expression of the receptor for advanced glycation endproducts (RAGE) is permissive for early pancreatic neoplasia. *Proc. Natl. Acad. Sci.*, 109, 18, 7031–7036, 2012.
59. Sun, Y., Harley, D., Vally, H., Sleigh, A., Impact of multi-drug resistance on tuberculosis recurrence and long-term outcome in China. *PLoS One*, 12, 1, e0168865, 2017 Jan 24.
60. Eum, K.H. and Lee, M., Targeting the autophagy pathway using ectopic expression of Beclin 1 in combination with rapamycin in drug-resistant v-Ha-ras-transformed NIH 3T3 cells. *Mol. Cells*, 31, 231–238, 2011.
61. Ge, J., Chen, Z., Huang, J., Chen, J., Yuan, W., Deng, Z., Chen, Z., Upregulation of autophagy-related gene-5 (ATG-5) is associated with chemoresistance in human gastric cancer. *PLoS One*, 9, 10, e110293, 2014.
62. Meschini, S., Condello, M., Calcabrini, A., Marra, M., Formisano, G., Lista, P., Arancia, G., The plant alkaloid voacamine induces apoptosis-independent autophagic cell death on both sensitive and multi-drug resistant human osteosarcoma cells. *Autophagy*, 4, 8, 1020–1033, 2008.
63. An, Y., Zhang, Z., Shang, Y., Jiang, X., Dong, J., Yu, P., Zhao, Q., miR-23b-3p regulates the chemoresistance of gastric cancer cells by targeting ATG12 and HMGB2. *Cell Death Dis.*, 6, 5, e1766–e1766, 2015.
64. O'Donovan, T.R., O'Sullivan, G.C., McKenna, S.L., Induction of autophagy by drug-resistant esophageal cancer cells promotes their survival and recovery following treatment with chemotherapeutics. *Autophagy*, 7, 5, 509–524, 2011.
65. Chittaranjan, S., Bortnik, S., Dragowska, W.H., Xu, J., Abeysundara, N., Leung, A., Gorski, S.M., Autophagy inhibition augments the anticancer effects of epirubicin treatment in anthracycline-sensitive and-resistant triple-negative breast cancerautophagy inhibition enhances efficacy of epirubicin in TNBC. *Clin. Cancer Res.*, 20, 12, 3159–3173, 2014.

66. Li, Y.J., Lei, Y.H., Yao, N. *et al.*, Autophagy and multi-drug resistance in cancer. *Chin J. Cancer*, 36, 52, 2017.
67. Lee, Y.J., Won, A.J., Lee, J., Jung, J.H., Yoon, S., Lee, B.M., Kim, H.S., Molecular mechanism of SAHA on regulation of autophagic cell death in tamoxifen-resistant MCF-7 breast cancer cells. *Int. J. Med. Sci.*, 9, 10, 881, 2012.
68. Hu, T., Wang, L., Zhang, L., Lu, L., Shen, J., Chan, R.L., Cho, C.H., Sensitivity of apoptosis-resistant colon cancer cells to tanshinones is mediated by autophagic cell death and p53-independent cytotoxicity. *Phytomedicine*, 22, 5, 536–544, 2015.
69. Aznar, M. Á., Lasa-Saracíbar, B., Blanco-Prieto, M.J., Edelfosine lipid nanoparticles overcome multi-drug resistance in K-562 leukemia cells by a caspase-independent mechanism. *Mol. Pharmaceutics*, 11, 8, 2650–2658, 2014.
70. Chiu, L.Y., Hu, M.E., Yang, T.Y., Hsin, I.L., Ko, J.L., Tsai, K.J., Sheu, G.T., Immunomodulatory protein from Ganoderma microsporum induces pro-death autophagy through Akt-mTOR-p70S6K pathway inhibition in multi-drug resistant lung cancer cells. *PLoS One*, 10, 5, e0125774, 2015.
71. Li, J.R., Cheng, C.L., Yang, C.R., Ou, Y.C., Wu, M.J., Ko, J.L., Dual inhibitor of phosphoinositide 3-kinase/mammalian target of rapamycin NVP-BEZ235 effectively inhibits cisplatin-resistant urothelial cancer cell growth through autophagic flux. *Toxicol. Lett.*, 220, 3, 267–276, 2013, doi: 10.1016/j.toxlet.2013.04.021.
72. Park, K.J., Lee, S.H., Kim, T.I., Lee, H.W., Lee, C.H., Kim, E.H., Kim, Y.S., A human scFv antibody against TRAIL receptor 2 induces autophagic cell death in both TRAIL-sensitive and TRAIL-resistant cancer cells. *Cancer Res.*, 67, 15, 7327–7334, 2007.
73. Wu, S., Wang, X., Chen, J., Chen, Y., Autophagy of cancer stem cells is involved with chemoresistance of colon cancer cells. *Biochem. Biophys. Res. Commun.*, 434, 4, 898–903, 2013.
74. Greene, L.M., Nolan, D.P., Regan-Komito, D., Campiani, G., Williams, D.C., Zisterer, D.M., Inhibition of late-stage autophagy synergistically enhances pyrrolo-1, 5-benzoxazepine-6-induced apoptotic cell death in human colon cancer cells. *Int. J. Oncol.*, 43, 3, 927–935, 2013.
75. Michel, V., Licon-Munoz, Y., Trujillo, K., Bisoffi, M., Parra, K.J., Inhibitors of vacuolar ATPase proton pumps inhibit human prostate cancer cell invasion and prostate-specific antigen expression and secretion. *Int. J. Cancer*, 132, 2, E1–E10, 2013.
76. Luo, S. and Rubinsztein, D.C., Apoptosis blocks Beclin 1-dependent autophagosome synthesis: An effect rescued by Bcl-xL. *Cell Death Differ.*, 17, 2, 268–277, 2010.
77. Kim, Y.S., Shin, J.H., Bae, M.K., Lee, C.Y., Kim, D.J., Chung, K.Y., Lee, J.G., Autophagy activity in pulmonary metastatic tumor tissues from colorectal cancer: A pilot study. *Yonsei Med. J.*, 55, 6, 1484–1488, 2014.
78. Cui, J., Hu, Y.F., Feng, X.M., Tian, T., Guo, Y.H., Ma, J.W., Zhang, H.Y., EGFR inhibitors and autophagy in cancer treatment. *Tumor Biol.*, 35, 11701–11709, 2014.

6

Transporter Inhibitors: A Chemotherapeutic Regimen to Improve the Clinical Outcome of Colorectal Cancer

Rishabha Malviya*, Arun Kumar Singh and Deepika Yadav

Abstract

Colorectal cancer treatment failures are mostly due to drug resistance, which is the primary cause of treatment failure (CRC). There are two types of resistance: primary and secondary (secondary resistance). Oncogenic stem cells, intratumor variability, the Warburg effect, and modifications to drug metabolism and drug target mutations are only a few of the processes that have been implicated in drug resistance. It is commonly accepted that the most frequent and early resistance mechanism is regulated by the ATP-binding cassette (ABC) transporter. Overexpression of the ABC transporter in drug-resistant cancer cells reduces the anticancer efficacy of both the conventional cytotoxic anticancer medications and the targeted chemotherapeutic agents widely used to treat CRC. Although there are few publications on the use of transporter inhibitors to reverse drug resistance in CRC, it is vital to recognize the relevance of drug resistance in solid tumors or the well-resistance reversing medicines seen in other tumor types. The pairing of ABC transporter inhibitors with chemotherapeutic medicines for resistance reversal has previously been studied in clinical trials without the selection of individuals whose tumors had a high expression of ABC transporters. Patients whose malignancies overexpress the ABC transporter may now be identified using tailored treatment. These individuals should get anticancer medications that do not act as transporter substrates. Chemotherapeutic regimens might also contain transporter inhibitors to enhance the clinical result.

Keywords: Colorectal cancer, chemotherapeutic agents, molecular targeted therapy, drug transporters, chemotherapy

**Corresponding author*: rishabhamalviya19@gmail.com

Rishabha Malviya, Arun Kumar Singh and Deepika Yadav. Multi-Drug Resistance in Cancer: Mechanism and Treatment Strategies, (105–130) © 2023 Scrivener Publishing LLC

6.1 Introduction

Among all cancers, colorectal cancer (CRC) is the third most frequently detected and the second leading cause of death [1]. Patients who have potentially curative surgery for early-stage colorectal cancer (CRC) are more likely to acquire the metastatic disease than those who do not. After a colectomy, patients may benefit from adjuvant chemotherapy to eliminate any remaining cancer cells and lower their risk of recurrence. Chemotherapy has a bad prognosis and response in more advanced diseases of CRC. Metastatic CRC has a 5-year survival rate of less than 10%. In order to come up with better treatment options, more basic and translational research is very necessary.

Depending on the tumor stage and patient features, there are a variety of treatment options for colorectal cancer (CRC). In the early stages of cancer, surgical resection is the most prevalent method of treatment. Polypectomy or trans-abdominal resection is employed depending on the location of the tumor and the level of invasion. Chemotherapy will be utilized as a preoperative treatment for advanced-stage CRC and as an adjuvant treatment for post-surgical recurrence prevention [2, 3]. 5-fluorouracil (5-FU), capecitabine, and other fluoropyrimidines are first-line chemotherapy treatments for metastatic colorectal cancer. With additional cytotoxic medicines such as irinotecan and oxaliplatin, they can produce an improved therapeutic response and prolonged progression-free survival [4]. FOLFOX, FOLFIRI, and FOLFOXIRI are among the most often used conventional chemotherapy regimens in clinics as are CAPOX (capecitabine and oxaliplatin) [2] and FOLFOXIRI [5-FU, leucovorin, oxaliplatin, and irinotecan]. In combination, the various anticancer medicines have separate modes of action and provide synergistic anticancer effects [5].

Molecular targeted therapy for metastatic CRC has been an important treatment option since the early 2000s. It has been shown that EGFR overexpression occurs in 65–70% of CRC tumors, and this has been linked to disease progression, a poor prognosis, and a shorter patient survival time [6]. Anti-EGFR monoclonal antibodies cetuximab and panitumumab have been authorized for use in clinical trials. Both as monotherapy and in conjunction with other chemotherapy regimens, they are employed in order to decrease the downstream signaling of ERK and Ras signaling pathways, which in turn slows cancer growth and survival [7, 8]. Additionally, the two EGFR monoclonal antibodies work better together than either one alone in terms of response and progression-free survival.

Bevacizumab, ramucirumab, and aflibercept are all monoclonal antibodies against the vascular endothelial growth factor (VEGF).

Angiogenesis and tumor growth are inhibited as a result of the decreased density and potency of the blood vessels feeding the malignancies. Trials on individuals with metastatic CRC found that VEGF monoclonal antibodies improved survival [9, 10].

In the last several years, immunotherapy has shown remarkable results in a wide range of cancers. Cancer cells that contain tumor-associated antigens are killed when the PD-1 and CLTA-1 coinhibitory molecules are inhibited, restoring T cell activation, stimulating the antitumor immune response, and stimulating antitumor immunity [11]. For CRC patients with MSI-H/dMMR tumors, immune checkpoint inhibitors have shown promising effectiveness [12], leading to the recent FDA approval of the PD-1 inhibitors (pembrolizumab and nivolumab) and the CLTA-4 inhibitor (ipilimumab).

6.2 CRC Transporters or ATP-Binding Cassette

6.2.1 ABC Transporter Family

ABC transporters are found in all living species, from microorganisms to humans, and represent a huge and ubiquitous class of proteins. They act as imports and exports of their substrates, depending on their needs. Eukaryotic ABC transporters are mostly exporters, but ABC transporters in prokaryotes may operate as importers [13]. Cellular concentrations of hormones, lipids, metabolites, pathogens and other small molecules may be controlled by pumping them out of cells across the cell membrane using ABC transporters in humans, which are energy-dependent efflux transporters. For substrate recognition and translocation, all ABC transporters have a core structure consisting of two transmembrane domains (TMDs), while the ATP binding domains (NBDs) supply energy. Homo- and heterodimerization of ABC transporters in eukaryotes may occur in either full or half-transporter forms, depending on how many ABC transporters are present on each polypeptide, respectively. Beginning in the year 2000, the ABC transporter names and numbers were standardized under a single nomenclature scheme. There are seven subfamilies of ABC transporter genes in this system, based on the similarity in gene structure and sequence homolog and order of the NBD/TMD sequences [14, 15].

6.2.2 ABC Transporters and CRC Initiation

Adenomas and adenocarcinomas are two of the most common types of cancer in the gastrointestinal tract, and it is commonly accepted that the progression from normal colon tissue to malignant tumors is a multi-step process [16, 17]. Several genetic alterations and/or epigenetic modifications are necessary for the growth of cancer. The processes driving the adenoma-carcinoma changeover in CRC development have been the subject of much inquiry.

Protecting the body against xenobiotic damage is a key function of the ABC transporters (such as P-gp, ABCG2, and MRPs), which are widely expressed on intestinal mucosal surfaces. Tumor start and development may be aided by the differential expression of these transporters in healthy vs malignant tissues, according to some research. ABC transporters have yet to have a definite role in the onset and development of colon cancer.

Micsik *et al.* used a fluorescence-based calcein transport assay to examine the functional activity of P-gp and MRP1 in newly separated colon cancer cells and healthy normal colon epithelial cells from surgical samples [18]. CRC cells had significantly lower P-gp transport activity compared to normal enterocytes, while MRP1 transport activity was not affected [18]. CRC risk was shown to be related to P-gp genetic variants that impair transport activity [19]. Colon adenomas (pedunculated polyps) have also been shown to have a decreased ABCG2 expression compared to the neighboring normal colon mucosa [20]. As a result, the development of colorectal cancer (CRC) may be facilitated. The ABCG2 expression in colon cancer has decreased similarly in two previous investigations [21, 22]. However, Calcagno *et al.* solely used GeneChip data from NCBI's GEO database to examine ABCG2 mRNA expression. Gupta *et al.* reported a limited sample size (n 14 13) and included patients who had previously had chemoradiation treatment. ABCG2 gene suppression has been linked to abnormal ABCG2 promoter methylation in a small number of cancers. Recent studies have shown that microRNAs can be used to methylate ABCG2 DNA in colon cancer cell lines and cancerous tissue from patients with colon cancer [23]. Gene promoter methylation may reduce ABCG2 expression throughout the carcinogenic process that leads to the development of colorectal cancer (CRC) (Figure 6.1).

It is well known that environmental variables have a role in tumor start and development [24], and this is particularly true for colorectal cancer. According to epidemiological and laboratory-based research, diet is a key component in the development of CRC [25, 26]. There are a number of recognized dietary carcinogens, such as benzo(a)pyrene conjugates, alfatoxin B1, N-nitroso compounds, and 2-amino-1methyl-6 phenylimidazo[4,5-b] pyridine (PhIP),

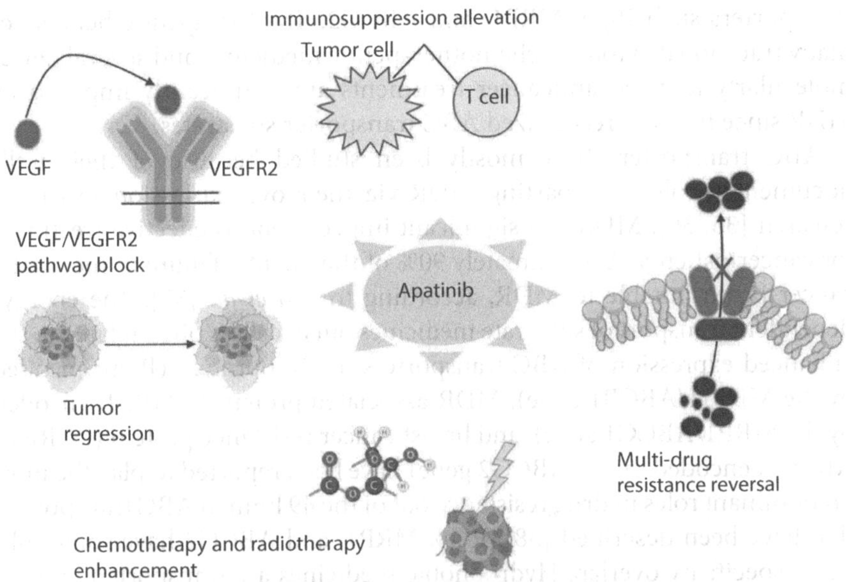

Figure 6.1 A diagram showing how ABCG2 overexpression contributes to MDR and how miR-519c/HuR offer potential therapeutic targets for bypassing ABCG2-mediated MDR in colorectal cancer.

that are linked to gene alterations that enable or accelerate the development of colorectal cancer (CRC) [27, 28]. Some xenobiotic transporters, notably ABCG2, have been shown to bind to these food-derived carcinogens [29].

IBD patients (including ulcerative colitis and Crohn's disease) have also been linked to a higher chance of developing colitis-associated CRC [30] because of chronic intestinal inflammation. These polyps have been shown to include an increased inflammatory microenvironment [31]. Mice with chronic inflammation developed colon cancer as a result of the DNA damage they suffered [32]. In ulcerative colitis patients with active inflammation, ABCG2 expression is lower than in those who are in remission [33]. Unfolded protein response (UPR) has been linked to decreased ABCG2 expression in IBD and altered ABCG2 transport function [34].

6.2.3 ABC Transporters and the Resistance of Cancer Cells to Chemotherapy

One of the biggest obstacles to cancer chemotherapy's success is multidrug resistance (MDR). There is a common mechanism for MDR that includes the efflux of anticancer medicines from cancer cells through ABC transporters such P-gp, MRP1, and ABCG2. The therapeutic benefits of many traditional cytotoxic chemotherapeutic medicines and several newer molecularly targeted anticancer treatments are significantly impeded by MDR since they are recognized ABC transporter substrates.

ABC transporters have mostly been studied because of their well-documented role in imparting MDR via their overexpression in cancer research [35, 36]. MDR is a significant impediment to effective treatment for cancer patients. Approximately 90% of therapeutic failure in metastatic cancer is attributable to MDR, according to Wu *et al.* [37]. The energy-dependent transport of substrate medicines out of cells is often related to the enhanced expression of ABC transporters. P-glycoprotein (P-gp, encoded by the MDR-1/ABCB1 gene), MDR-associated protein 1 (MRP1, encoded by the MRP1/ABCC1 gene), and breast cancer resistance protein (BCRP or ABCG2, encoded by the ABCG2 gene) have been reported to play the most predominant roles in drug resistance out of the 49 human ABC transporters that have been described [38]. P-gp, MRP1, and ABCG2 have some substrate specificity overlap. Hydrophobic medicines are transported by P-gp and MRP1 whereas organic anionic compounds are transported by MRP1 (conjugated to glutathione or glucuronate). Drugs including methotrexate, mitoxantrone, and anthracyclines may be transported via ABCG2 [39].

Among the ABC transporters that provide MDR to cancer cells is ABCB1 (MDR1/P-glycoprotein/P-gp). In polarized cells, P-gp is found on the apical or luminal membranes. Brush boundary membrane, biliary canalicular membrane of hepatocytes, luminal epithelium of proximal tubule epithelial cells of the kidney, and endothelial cells of the blood-brain barrier all include it. P-gp plays a critical role in protecting these biological barriers from harmful chemicals and metabolites [40]. The MDR phenotype is conferred to cancer cells by this transporter because of its high transport capacity and wide substrate recognition by P-gp. The apical surfaces of the superficial columnar epithelial cells of the colon in the gastrointestinal tract are abundantly expressed for P-gp [41]. In terms of colorectal carcinogenesis and tumor grade, P-gp has been linked [42].

On the basis of MDR that was not connected with P-gp, ABCC1/MRP1 originally became known [43]. It gives resistance to hydrophobic anticancer drugs, such P-gp.

Further functional characterization of MRP1 revealed that its preferred substrates are organic anions such as glutathione or anticancer medicines conjugated with sulphate [44]. Anions that are unconjugated and free glutathione may also be transported by MRP1 [45].

Initially, ABCG2 was reported to be a half-transporter in MDR cancers that did not express either P-gp or MRP1 [46]. ABCG2 is likewise a high-capacity drug efflux transporter with broad substrate specificity. For example, 5-FU, irinotecan, mitoxantrone, and topotecan are among the most regularly used regimens for the treatment of colorectal cancer (CRC) when ABCG2 expression is elevated [47]. Chemically unrelated substances are aggressively expelled from cells by this enzyme.

MDR conferred by ABC transporters other than ABCA1 has also been identified in CRC. 5-FU's monophosphorylated metabolite may be transported by MRP5, which also promotes cross-resistance to oxaliplatin and antifolates in patients with colon cancer [48]. Celecoxib has been demonstrated to increase the expression of MRP4 and MRP5 in colon cancer cells in a cell line investigation [49]. Celecoxib, 5-FU and irinotecan were shown to have a poor anticancer response rate in clinical studies in which patients were given the combination of these medications [49]; this is consistent with this conclusion. During colon carcinogenesis, Wnt signaling was shown to suppress ABCC3 in recent research that compared colon cancer tissue with normal tissue and colon cancer cell lines. Etoposide and teniposide have been demonstrated to increase ABCC3 expression and give acquired drug resistance in colon cancer cell lines [50].

Besides the function ABC transporters play in regulating MDR, ABCG2 is also a survival factor for cancer stem cells (CSCs) [51]. "CSCs" refers to a subset of cancer cells having stem cell traits (such as self-renewal and tumorigenicity) and the ability to differentiate into many cell lines. Chemoresistance in this population is thought to remain in tumors, where it may lead to recurrence and metastasis via the development of new cancers [52]. Anticancer medicines, according to the CSC hypothesis, must eliminate all remaining CSCs if they are to have a long-lasting effect. In primary human colorectal tumor samples [53, 54] and CRC cell lines [55], CSCs have been found. CD133-positive human CRC cells' self-renewal and chemoresistance depend on ABCG2 [56], according to a recent study. MDR cancer cells and CSCs might be targeted using drugs that target ABCG2. A novel target for the therapy of colon cancer has been identified as colon CSCs [57].

6.3 Clinical Evidence for the Function of ABC Transporters in CRC MDR

6.3.1 Intrinsic Drug Resistance in Colon Cancer Upregulation of P-gp at Detection

Over half of all human malignancies are thought to express P-gp to such a high degree that it confers treatment resistance [58]. Most chemotherapeutic drugs fail to work in colon cancer, making it a notoriously difficult malignancy to treat. A high P-gp expression has been found at the time of diagnosis for colorectal cancer (CRC), which has been linked to the inherent resistance of various colon cancer cell lines accessible in the cancer research community [59–61]. Chemotherapeutic drugs may also increase the expression of P-gp in cancer cells. P-gp is upregulated in colon cancer cells via a variety of signaling mechanisms. As a master regulator of hypoxic gene response in malignancies, hypoxia-inducible factor-1 alpha (HIF-1) has been found in human colon cancer cell lines to promote the high expression of P-gp [62]. The suppression of HIF-1 in LoVo multicellular spheroids has been shown to reverse drug resistance by downregulating P-gp [63]. There is evidence that NF-kB activation induces P-gp expression in the HCT15 colon cancer cell line, and that blocking NF-kB may enhance daunomycin's apoptotic impact by decreasing P-gp expression [64].

It is thought that a subset of cancer cells inside a tumor is responsible for tumor development, resistance to treatment, and recurrence [65]. CSC-rich cell subpopulations may be identified by the expression of the CD133 antigen in a variety of tumors, including CRC. For the first time, it has been shown that fresh colon tumor specimens of the varied stage of the disease include CD133-positive cells, which have the capacity for the growth and formation of tumor spheres [56]. These CRC tumor tissues had ABCG2- and CD133-positive cells expressed, as shown by immunofluorescence analysis [56]. More notably, suppressing ABCG2 in CD133-positive CRC cells and another colon cancer cell line LS174T greatly increased the effectiveness of chemotherapy (5-FU and oxaliplatin) caused apoptosis in experimental NOD/SCID mice [56].

6.3.2 Proliferating Tumor Cells Have MRP1 on Their Surface

The cancer cells that are discharged into the bloodstream of cancer patients by their main tumor are referred to as circulating tumor cells (CTC) [66]. It has been suggested that CTCs are multifunctional biomarkers that make it easier to track the course of the tumor during therapy. CTCs have also been linked to distant metastases, according to reports. Different kinds of tumors have been reported to have poor PFS and overall survival (OS) when CTC levels are high [67].

As a member of the ABC transporter superfamily, MRP1 facilitates the efflux of a broad variety of anticancer medicines (including folate-based antimetabolites, anthracyclines, cytotoxic alkaloids, camptothecins, and antiandrogen) and protects cancer cells from cytotoxic effects [68].

Metastatic CRC patients with MRP1-positive CTCs had a substantially worse PFS (2.1 months vs 9.1 months; P 14.003) when treated with irinotecan-based chemotherapy, compared to those with MRP1-negative CTCs [69].

Nuclear hormone receptor superfamily member PXR is a ligand-activated transcription factor [70]. Several kinds of cancer, including colon cancer, have been linked to increased PXR expression. As a result, the clearance of drugs from the body is altered by the activation of several drug-metabolizing enzymes and drug transporters. Chemoresistant CRC cells with elevated MRP3 mRNA expression have been linked to PXR over-expression [71].

Two separate TCGA cohorts found a significant (P 14.0023) positive connection between MRP3 and PXR expression [72]. For stage I and II CRC patients, this is a substantial risk factor for poor survival [73]. It was shown that PXR transcriptionally stimulates MRP3 by binding directly to its promoter, increasing the efflux of the MRP3-substrate anticancer drug (oxaliplatin), and mediating drug resistance [73].

6.4 General Approaches

Chemotherapy for cancer patients must address the MDR issue. Developing novel anticancer medications that do not interact with ABC transporters is a sensible approach to MDR since ABC transporters recognize and expel anticancer drugs. Since anticancer medications must breach the plasma membrane to enter cells and MDR transporters have extraordinarily wide substrate specificities, this appears to be a distant possibility.

In addition to epothilones and second/third generation taxanes, new inhibitors of topoisomerase I/II have been developed that have a lower molecular affinity for P-gp [74]. Microtubule-targeting sagopilone (ZK-EPO) is an epothilone B derivative intended to be a poor P-gp substrate [75]. Compared to previous microtubule-targeting drugs, its anticancer efficacy was shown to be much less influenced by P-gp overexpression [76, 77].

Tyrosine kinase inhibitors (TKIs), which are well-known as ABC transporter substrates, have been conjugated with platinum-based medicines by the research team using a hybrid drug design technique [78]. This strategy turns TKIs into nonsubstrates rather than substrates for the ABC transporter, hence avoiding transporter-mediated resistance. ABC transporters at the blood-brain barrier prevent TKIs from penetrating the brain to treat metastases. A study in BALB/c mice found that the hybrids were able to evade drug efflux via the transporters, accumulating more than the original TKI in the brain. New medications for the treatment of colorectal cancer (CRC) might benefit from a similar approach. It is also possible to find MDR-modifying drugs that block the MDR transporters in a competitive or noncompetitive way. Preventing cancer cells from extruding transporter substrate medicines is likely to increase the anticancer impact of these MDR-modifying medications an anticancer medication that binds to P-gp and blocks P-gp-mediated protein efflux was found to boost intracellular concentrations of anticancer drugs in multi-drug-resistant cells in the 1980s [79]. MDR may be reversed by blocking efflux transporters, which reinforced the belief that MDR could be reversed. A variety of P-gp inhibitors have been discovered [80] to enhance chemotherapy for multidrug-resistant cancers, and various clinical studies have been conducted to test this MDR reversal theory. Drugs that might be used in the clinic based on recognized medical reasons and were shown to be P-gp inhibitors in the laboratory were used in these studies. However, *in vivo*, these medicines were only marginally effective as P-gp antagonists. As a result, it was impossible to establish a conclusive link between the improvement in therapeutic response and the reduction of P-gp-mediated resistance in the studies that were not structured and randomized. As a result, the combined use of these inhibitors with anticancer medicines was limited by poor effectiveness and excessive toxicity at acceptable levels. As new P-gp inhibitors entered the market, it was discovered that several of them interfered with cytochrome P450, reducing their efficacy [81]. It was decided to end an important phase III Cancer and Leukemia Group B (CALGB) trial early due to excessive mortality in the experimental arm during treatment initiation (valspodar, 2nd generation P-gp inhibitor) in previously untreated AML patients [82]. Toxicities halted two other large phase III trials in NSCLC patients using a third-generation P-gp inhibitor (tariquidar) and first-line chemotherapy [83, 84].

Since MDR transporter inhibitors have a wide range of bioactivities and can cause a variety of undesirable side effects, clinical trials to convert them into therapeutics have been fruitless. To test the MDR reversal hypothesis and avoid drug resistance in anticancer therapy, it's important to create potent MDR inhibitors with no other biological activities. This led researchers to look for other drug transporters and their inhibitors that are involved in the development of MDR cells with reduced drug accumulation.

In light of the growing evidence that additional ABC transporter family members (e.g. MRP1 and ABCG2) play an important role in MDR, antagonists that can block multiple transporters have to be developed. The variety of inhibitors that have been discovered so far is astounding. However, there is no unambiguous structure-function link that can explain the definite needs of an inhibitor. The inhibition of P-gp and ABCG2 was also sought to boost oral bioavailability and brain penetration of their substrate medicines, in addition to their role in anticancer drug resistance. Elacridar, an ABCG2 inhibitor, has been demonstrated to increase the oral bioavailability of topotecan in humans [85]. A mouse model and pediatric patients both showed improved oral bioavailability and anticancer efficacy of irinotecan when given in combination with gefitinib [86, 87]. Topotecan's brain penetration was increased by gefitinib's inhibition of P-gp and/or ABCG2 [88], underscoring the need for powerful inhibitors of these two transporters.

6.5 By Blocking Tyrosine Kinase Inhibitors from Inhibiting MDR Transporters

In addition to CML, lung, breast, and colon cancers, TKIs represent a novel family of molecularly targeted cancer chemotherapeutic drugs. They control downstream signaling pathways involved in cancer proliferation, invasion, metastasis, and angiogenesis by competing with the ATP-binding site of the catalytic domain of numerous oncogenic tyrosine kinases. Several ABC transporters, including P-gp, ABCG2, and perhaps others, have been shown to be potently and specifically inhibited by TKIs in recent years, reigniting interest in the development of drug transporter inhibitors to evade MDR. Inhibition of P-gp and/or ABCG2 by imatinib, the first TKI authorized for CML, has been proven to reverse MDR [89, 90]. In different *in vitro* and *in vivo* settings, several additional TKIs have been shown to overcome drug resistance that is mediated by MDR transporters. These include but are not limited to the following: osimertinib, pelitinib, vandetanib, vatalanib, ceritinib, and apatinib [91]. ABC transporters are upregulated in the hypoxic cancer microenvironment, which reduces medication response through many mechanisms, including hypoxia.

However, a new TKI (vatalanib) has been shown to selectively sensitize ABCB1 and ABCG2-overexpressing MDR colon cancer cells to chemotherapy under hypoxia [92].

TKIs have shown promise MDR reversal activity, although the structure-activity link for the ABC transporter inhibitory impact of TKIs is still not very well understood [93, 94].

TKIs have been shown to bypass MDR in both *in vitro* and *in vivo*, however, only a few clinical trials have shown the potentiation of chemotherapeutic medicines' anticancer effects (Table 6.1) [95]. Although none

Table 6.1 Clinical trials showing potential chemotherapeutic medicines anticancer effect.

Combined treatment	Kind of cancer	The identifier for clinical trials/phase of a clinical trial
Masitinib + FOLFIRI	CRC that has spread to other parts of the body	NCT03556956/phase 2,3
Nintedanib + Capecitabine	CRC that has spread throughout the body metastatic	NCT02393755/phase 2
Erlotinib + Topotecan	Tumors that are hard to remove	NCT00611468/phase 1
Regorafenib + Capecitabine + Radiotherapy	Acquired recurrence of rectal cancer	NCT02910843/phase 1

of these studies was focused on ABC transporter-mediated MDR reversal, they were undertaken in a variety of tumor types, not only colorectal cancer.

6.6 Components Produced from Natural Sources that Inhibit MDR Transporters

Human trials of the first three generations of P-gp inhibitors have been disappointing because of their toxicities at the transporter-modifying concentrations [96–98]. Plant-derived materials are now being considered by researchers in their search for better P-gp inhibitors that are both safer and more effective. The anticancer effects of other concurrently administered chemotherapy drugs have been shown to be improved by the inhibition of P-gp by a variety of alkaloids, flavonoids, and other plant constituents [99–101]. (i) Diosmin, glabridin, kaempferid, quercetin, and apigenin are ABCB1 inhibitors; (ii) apigenin; kaempferol; and myricetin are ABCC1 inhibitors; and (iii) daidzein; silymarin; and hesperidin are ABCG2 inhibitors [102, 103]. For the treatment of colorectal cancer, Lee *et al.* recently published a comprehensive review of the identification of P-gp inhibitors and MDR reversal agents from herbal compounds [104]. For most studies, researchers used the Caco-2 cell line, which is well-known for expressing high levels of P-gp and developing microvilli on the apical surface [105–108]. Animal studies have been few and far between [109–112]. Herbal compounds have not been tested on humans in any of these studies on MDR reversal. Further research is needed to determine the optimal dose schedules for MDR transporter inhibition for these natural source transporter inhibitors since oral administration is expected [102]. After oral intake of flavonoid metabolite, the pharmacokinetics, bioavailability and activity of the flavonoid metabolites should also be investigated [113, 114].

6.7 Inhibiting ABC Transporters in Other Ways for CRC MDR Circumvention

Hypoxia promotes the transcription of several hypoxia-inducible genes via the master oxygen homeostasis regulator HIF-1. HIF-1 and MDR1 mRNA expressions were observed to be greater in CRC cells under hypoxia settings than under normoxic conditions [62]. For the four primary anticancer medications used in the treatment of colon cancer (i.e. 5-FU, irinotecan, vincristine, and doxorubicin), the cytotoxic impact of hypoxic conditions was significantly decreased in the LoVo model [63]. Silencing HIF-1 was shown to restore the LoVo cell model's sensitivity to all four chemotherapeutic agents [63]. The HIF-1(+)/P-gp(+) patient group was also shown to be more resistant to 5-FU-based chemotherapy than the HIF-1 (+)/P-gp (+) patient population [63].

mRNA degradation and translation inhibition may be induced by miRNAs, which are short noncoding RNAs that form imperfect hybrids with the 30 untranslated regions (30 UTR) of the mRNAs they target. Some miRNAs (miR-520h, -519c, -328, -181a, and -487a) that target ABCG2 have been discovered by researchers [115].

We also found that in ABCG2-overexpressing resistant CRC cell line models, the ABCG2 30 UTR was shortened [116]. ABCG2 repression is exacerbated by this 30 UTR truncation, which reduces the miR-519c binding site and its repressive effects on ABCG2. A new indirect mechanism through which low levels of miR-519c stimulate upregulation of the mRNA-binding protein HuR and ultimately lead to ABCG2 overexpression and enhanced resistance has been discovered by our research in addition to the direct regulation of ABCG2 by miR-519c. By increasing their stability and/or translation, HuR modulates AU-rich mRNA, which has been widely researched [117]. The high levels of HuR/ABCG2 in tumors and the poor response of patients to chemotherapy were shown to be related to the recent investigation of colon cancer tissues and their matched neighboring noncancerous colon [118]. MiR-519c and the HuR inhibitor are thus potential tools for reducing ABCG2 and eliminating MDR in CRC. A depiction of ABCG2's role in MDR and how miR-519c/HuR are new therapeutic targets for overcoming ABCG2-mediated MDR in CRC is shown in Figure 6.1.

6.8 Challenges and Future Prospective

Since the last decade has seen a lot of research on ABC transporters' role in MDR, the clinical value of modulating the transporters to overcome MDR has not yet been established. The assessment of P-gp expression (and other main MDR transporters) makes it difficult to evaluate the importance of transporter overexpression in clinical drug resistance [119–125]. In recent years, researchers have worked to improve the accuracy of methods for detecting biological samples' levels of ABC transporter. PET imaging in patients with MDR1-expressing tumors before and after an MDR1 inhibitor was administered to patients with radiolabelled substrates, e.g. sestamibi, which targeted ABC transporters in human malignancies [126]. In clinical trials, patients with MDR tumors may have a better chance of responding to drug efflux transporter inhibitors if the method can be refined further. To understand the function of MDR transporters in drug resistance, sensitive, repeatable, and validated methods for identifying transporter expressions in malignancies must be established. It is critical to plan clinical trials that focus on ABC transporter inhibition as a means of reversing MDR. MDR reversal was first tested on patients with acute lymphoblastic leukemia [82]. No clinical trials using ABC transporter inhibitors in combination with chemotherapeutic drugs for MDR reversal in CRC have been performed to our knowledge. Trials in humans should be conducted to determine which subsets of patients are most likely to benefit from the ABC transporter inhibitor and chemotherapeutic drugs being tested. In order to provide patients with the best possible treatment, it is necessary to identify biomarkers that can predict how well a patient will respond to a drug combination. Biomarkers that accurately predict treatment response are lacking in the CRC field. While the lack of response to 5-FU therapy is predicted by mismatch repair deficiency (dMMR), the increased response to pembrolizumab is suggested by dMMR [127]. KRAS/NRAS/BRAF mutations are the only biomarkers that indicate a lack of response to anti-EGFR treatment in CRC and, as a result, are a contraindication [128].

In vitro, many novel targeted drugs are ABC transporter substrates. P-gp and other ABC transporters may not be relevant to clinical resistance to targeted agents such as neratinib, regorafenib, or vemurafenib, which are emerging TKIs in the treatment of metastatic colorectal cancer.

6.9 Conclusion

The MDR reversal hypothesis has been reexamined by the cancer research community in light of the recent discoveries of safer and more selective MDR transporter inhibitors and the increasing ability to identify overexpression of ABC transporters in tumor tissues *in situ*. Poor clinical outcomes in CRC patients are shown to be associated with the overexpression of the ABC transporter, as has been seen in many other forms of cancers as well. To successfully employ transporter inhibitors to overcome MDR, it is important to understand how critical MDR is in solid tumors and how well-known MDR-reversing drugs have been discovered in other tumor types. Patients with malignancies that expressed high levels of ABC transporter expression were not selected for clinical studies using the combination of ABC transporter inhibitors and chemotherapeutic medicines to reverse MDR. Patients whose malignancies overexpress ABC transporters may be identified in the age of personalized medicine in order to optimize treatment selection and clinical outcome. In the therapeutic environment, even if ABC transporter inhibitors do not increase anticancer therapy response, they may be useful biomarkers for predicting clinical response to certain medications.

References

1. Gill, S., Thomas, R.R., Goldberg, R.M., Review article: Colorectal cancer chemotherapy. *Aliment. Pharmacol. Ther.*, 18, 683–692, 2003.
2. Hu, T., Li, L.F., Shen, J., Zhang, L., Cho, C.H., Chronic inflammation and colorectal cancer: The role of vascular endothelial growth factor. *Curr. Pharm. Des.*, 21, 2960–2967, 2015.
3. Li, L.F., Chan, R.L., Lu, L., Shen, J., Zhang, L., Wu, W.K., Wang, L., Hu, T., Li, M.X., Cho, C.H., Cigarette smoking and gastrointestinal diseases: The causal relationship and underlying molecular mechanisms (review). *Int. J. Mol. Med.*, 34, 372–380, 2014.

4. Stein, A., Atanackovic, D., Bokemeyer, C., Current standards and new trends in the primary treatment of colorectal cancer. *Eur. J. Cancer*, 47, Suppl 3, S312–S314, 2011.
5. Cunningham, D., Atkin, W., Lenz, H.J., Lynch, H.T., Minsky, B., Nordlinger, B., Starling, N., Colorectal cancer. *Lancet*, 375, 1030–1047, 2010.
6. Dallas, N.A., Xia, L., Fan, F., Gray, M.J., Gaur, P., van Buren, G., Samuel, S., Kim, M.P., Lim, S.J., Ellis, L.M., Chemoresistant colorectal cancer cells, the cancer stem cell phenotype, and increased sensitivity to insulin-like growth factor-I receptor inhibition. *Cancer Res.*, 69, 1951–1957, 2009.
7. White, N.J., Delaying antimalarial drug resistance with combination chemotherapy. *Parassitologia*, 41, 301–308, 1999.
8. Juliano, R.L. and Ling, V., A surface glycoprotein modulating drug permeability in Chinese hamster ovary cell mutants. *Biochim. Biophys. Acta*, 455, 152–162, 1976.
9. Thomas, H. and Coley, H.M., Overcoming multi-drug resistance in cancer: An update on the clinical strategy of inhibiting p-glycoprotein. *Cancer Control*, 10, 159–165, 2003.
10. Holohan, C., Van Schaeybroeck, S., Longley, D.B., Johnston, P.G., Cancer drug resistance: An evolving paradigm. *Nat. Rev. Cancer*, 13, 714–726, 2013.
11. Krishna, R. and Mayer, L.D., Multi-drug resistance (MDR) in cancer. Mechanisms, reversal using modulators of MDR and the role of MDR modulators in influencing the pharmacokinetics of anticancer drugs. *Eur. J. Pharm. Sci.*, 11, 265–283, 2000.
12. Gottesman, M.M., Fojo, T., Bates, S.E., Multi-drug resistance in cancer: Role of ATP-dependent transporters. *Nat. Rev. Cancer*, 2, 48–58, 2002.
13. Giacomini, K.M., Huang, S.M., Tweedie, D.J., Benet, L.Z., Brouwer, K.L., Chu, X., Dahlin, A., Evers, R., Fischer, V., Hillgren, K.M. *et al.*, Membrane transporters in drug development. *Nat. Rev. Drug Discovery*, 9, 215–236, 2010.
14. Duan, H., Hu, T., Foti, R.S., Pan, Y., Swaan, P.W., Wang, J., Potent and selective inhibition of plasma membrane monoamine transporter by HIV protease inhibitors. *Drug Metab. Dispos.*, 43, 1773–1780, 2015.
15. Szakács, G., Paterson, J.K., Ludwig, J.A., Booth-Genthe, C., Gottesman, M.M., Targeting multi-drug resistance in cancer. *Nat. Rev. Drug Discovery*, 5, 219–234, 2006.
16. Sharom, F.J., Shedding light on drug transport: Structure and function of the P-glycoprotein multi-drug transporter (ABCB1). *Biochem. Cell Biol.*, 84, 979–992, 2006.
17. Ward, A.B., Szewczyk, P., Grimard, V., Lee, C.W., Martinez, L., Doshi, R., Caya, A., Villaluz, M., Pardon, E., Cregger, C. *et al.*, Structures of P-glycoprotein reveal its conformational flexibility and an epitope on the nucleotide-binding domain. *Proc. Natl. Acad. Sci. U.S.A.*, 110, 13386–13391, 2013.
18. Slot, A.J., Molinski, S.V., Cole, S.P., Mammalian multi-drug-resistance proteins (MRPs). *Essays Biochem.*, 50, 179–207, 2011.

19. McDevitt, C.A., Collins, R.F., Conway, M., Modok, S., Storm, J., Kerr, I.D., Ford, R.C., Callaghan, R., Purification and 3D structural analysis of oligomeric human multi-drug transporter ABCG2. *Structure*, 14, 1623–1632, 2006.
20. Liu, Z., Qiu, M., Tang, Q.L., Liu, M., Lang, N., Bi, F., Establishment and biological characteristics of oxaliplatin-resistant human colon cancer cell lines. *Chin. J. Cancer*, 29, 661–667, 2010.
21. Ekblad, L., Kjellström, J., Johnsson, A., Reduced drug accumulation is more important in acquired resistance against oxaliplatin than against cisplatin in isogenic colon cancer cells. *Anticancer Drugs*, 21, 523–531, 2010.
22. Yuan, J., Lv, H., Peng, B., Wang, C., Yu, Y., He, Z., Role of BCRP as a biomarker for predicting resistance to 5-fluorouracil in breast cancer. *Cancer Chemother. Pharmacol.*, 63, 1103–1110, 2009.
23. Fu, D. and Arias, I.M., Intracellular trafficking of P-glycoprotein. *Int. J. Biochem. Cell Biol.*, 44, 461–464, 2012.
24. Spoelstra, E.C., Dekker, H., Schuurhuis, G.J., Broxterman, H.J., Lankelma, J., P-glycoprotein drug efflux pump involved in the mechanisms of intrinsic drug resistance in various colon cancer cell lines. Evidence for a saturation of active daunorubicin transport. *Biochem. Pharmacol.*, 41, 349–359, 1991.
25. Fojo, A.T., Ueda, K., Slamon, D.J., Poplack, D.G., Gottesman, M.M., Pastan, I., Expression of a multi-drug-resistance gene in human tumors and tissues. *Proc. Natl. Acad. Sci. U.S.A.*, 84, 265–269, 1987.
26. Meschini, S., Calcabrini, A., Monti, E., Del Bufalo, D., Stringaro, A., Dolfini, E., Arancia, G., Intracellular P-glycoprotein expression is associated with the intrinsic multi-drug resistance phenotype in human colon adenocarcinoma cells. *Int. J. Cancer*, 87, 615–628, 2000.
27. Burger, H., van Tol, H., Brok, M., Wiemer, E.A., de Bruijn, E.A., Guetens, G., de Boeck, G., Sparreboom, A., Verweij, J., Nooter, K., Chronic imatinib mesylate exposure leads to reduced intracellular drug accumulation by induction of the ABCG2 (BCRP) and ABCB1 (MDR1) drug transport pumps. *Cancer Biol. Ther.*, 4, 747–752, 2005.
28. Bentires-Alj, M., Barbu, V., Fillet, M., Chariot, A., Relic, B., Jacobs, N., Gielen, J., Merville, M.P., Bours, V., NF-kappaB transcription factor induces drug resistance through MDR1 expression in cancer cells. *Oncogene*, 22, 90–97, 2003.
29. Ding, Z., Yang, L., Xie, X., Xie, F., Pan, F., Li, J., He, J., Liang, H., Expression and significance of hypoxia-inducible factor-1 alpha and MDR1/P-glycoprotein in human colon carcinoma tissue and cells. *J. Cancer Res. Clin. Oncol.*, 136, 1697–1707, 2010.
30. Chen, J., Ding, Z., Peng, Y., Pan, F., Li, J., Zou, L., Zhang, Y., Liang, H., HIF-1α inhibition reverses multi-drug resistance in colon cancer cells via downregulation of MDR1/P-glycoprotein. *PLoS One*, 9, e98882, 2014.
31. Wang, T., Chen, Z., Zhu, Y., Pan, Q., Liu, Y., Qi, X., Jin, L., Jin, J., Ma, X., Hua, D., Inhibition of transient receptor potential channel 5 reverses

5-Fluorouracil resistance in human colorectal cancer cells. *J. Biol. Chem.*, 290, 448–456, 2015.

32. Meijer, G.A., Schroeijers, A.B., Flens, M.J., Meuwissen, S.G., van der Valk, P., Baak, J.P., Scheper, R.J., Increased expression of multi-drug resistance related proteins Pgp, MRP1, and LRP/MVP occurs early in colorectal carcinogenesis. *J. Clin. Pathol.*, 52, 450–454, 1999.
33. Klappe, K., Hinrichs, J.W., Kroesen, B.J., Sietsma, H., Kok, J.W., MRP1 and glucosylceramide are coordinately over expressed and enriched in rafts during multi-drug resistance acquisition in colon cancer cells. *Int. J. Cancer*, 110, 511–522, 2004.
34. Tatebe, S., Sinicrope, F.A., Kuo, M.T., Induction of multi-drug resistance proteins MRP1 and MRP3 and gamma-glutamylcysteine synthetase gene expression by nonsteroidal anti-inflammatory drugs in human colon cancer cells. *Biochem. Biophys. Res. Commun.*, 290, 1427–1433, 2002.
35. Jendzelovský, R., Mikes, J., Koval', J., Soucek, K., Procházková, J., Kello, M., Sacková, V., Hofmanová, J., Kozubík, A., Fedorocko, P., Drug efflux transporters, MRP1 and BCRP, affect the outcome of hypericin-mediated photodynamic therapy in HT-29 adenocarcinoma cells. *Photochem. Photobiol. Sci.*, 8, 1716–1723, 2009.
36. Lv, Y., Zhao, S., Han, J., Zheng, L., Yang, Z., Zhao, L., Hypoxia-inducible factor-1α induces multi-drug resistance protein in colon cancer. *Onco Targets Ther.*, **8**, 1941–1948, 2015.
37. Ikegami, Y., Tatebe, S., Lin-Lee, Y.C., Xie, Q.W., Ishikawa, T., Kuo, M.T., Induction of MRP1 and gamma-glutamylcysteine synthetase gene expression by interleukin 1beta is mediated by nitric oxide-related signalings in human colorectal cancer cells. *J. Cell. Physiol.*, 185, 293–301, 2000.
38. Miyake, K., Mickley, L., Litman, T., Zhan, Z., Robey, R., Cristensen, B., Brangi, M., Greenberger, L., Dean, M., Fojo, T. *et al.*, Molecular cloning of cDNAs which are highly overexpressed in mitoxantrone-resistant cells: Demonstration of homology to ABC transport genes. *Cancer Res.*, 59, 8–13, 1999.
39. Ross, D.D., Yang, W., Abruzzo, L.V., Dalton, W.S., Schneider, E., Lage, H., Dietel, M., Greenberger, L., Cole, S.P., Doyle, L.A., Atypical multi-drug resistance: Breast cancer resistance protein messenger RNA expression in mitoxantrone-selected cell lines. *J. Natl. Cancer Inst.*, 91, 429–433, 1999.
40. Jung, K.A., Choi, B.H., Kwak, M.K., The c-MET/PI3K signaling is associated with cancer resistance to doxorubicin and photodynamic therapy by elevating BCRP/ABCG2 expression. *Mol. Pharmacol.*, 87, 465–476, 2015.
41. Zhu, M.M., Tong, J.L., Xu, Q., Nie, F., Xu, X.T., Xiao, S.D., Ran, Z.H., Increased JNK1 signaling pathway is responsible for ABCG2-mediated multi-drug resistance in human colon cancer. *PLoS One*, 7, e41763, 2012.
42. Herraez, E., Gonzalez-Sanchez, E., Vaquero, J., Romero, M.R., Serrano, M.A., Marin, J.J., Briz, O., Cisplatin-induced chemoresistance in colon cancer cells

involves FXR-dependent and FXR-independent up-regulation of ABC proteins. *Mol. Pharmacol.*, 9, 2565–2576, 2012.
43. Erlichman, C., Boerner, S.A., Hallgren, C.G., Spieker, R., Wang, X.Y., James, C.D., Scheffer, G.L., Maliepaard, M., Ross, D.D., Bible, K.C. *et al.*, The HER tyrosine kinase inhibitor CI1033 enhances cytotoxicity of 7-ethyl-10-hydroxycamptothecin and topotecan by inhibiting breast cancer resistance protein-mediated drug efflux. *Cancer Res.*, 61, 739–748, 2001.
44. Chikazawa, N., Tanaka, H., Tasaka, T., Nakamura, M., Tanaka, M., Onishi, H., Katano, M., Inhibition of Wnt signaling pathway decreases chemotherapy-resistant side-population colon cancer cells. *Anticancer Res.*, 30, 2041–2048, 2010.
45. Wilson, B.J., Schatton, T., Zhan, Q., Gasser, M., Ma, J., Saab, K.R., Schanche, R., Waaga-Gasser, A.M., Gold, J.S., Huang, Q. *et al.*, ABCB5 identifies a therapy-refractory tumor cell population in colorectal cancer patients. *Cancer Res.*, 71, 5307–5316, 2011.
46. Hinoshita, E., Uchiumi, T., Taguchi, K., Kinukawa, N., Tsuneyoshi, M., Maehara, Y., Sugimachi, K., Kuwano, M., Increased expression of an ATP-binding cassette superfamily transporter, multi-drug resistance protein 2, in human colorectal carcinomas. *Clin. Cancer Res.*, 6, 2401–2407, 2000.
47. Gradilone, A., Pulcinelli, F.M., Lotti, L.V., Trifirò, E., Martino, S., Gandini, O., Gianni, W., Frati, L., Aglianò, A.M., Gazzaniga, P., Celecoxib upregulates multi-drug resistance proteins in colon cancer: Lack of synergy with standard chemotherapy. *Curr. Cancer Drug Targets*, 8, 414–420, 2008.
48. Gillet, J.P. and Gottesman, M.M., Mechanisms of multi-drug resistance in cancer. *Methods Mol. Biol.*, 596, 47–76, 2010.
49. Wu, Y., Zhang, Y., Zhang, W., Sun, C., Wu, J., Tang, J., Reversing of multi-drug resistance breast cancer by co-delivery of P-gp siRNA and doxorubicin via folic acid-modified core-shell nanomicelles. *Colloids Surf. B Biointerfaces*, 138, 60–69, 2016.
50. Xie, N., Mou, L., Yuan, J., Liu, W., Deng, T., Li, Z., Jing, Y., Hu, Z., Modulating drug resistance by targeting BCRP/ABCG2 using retrovirus-mediated RNA interference. *PLoS One*, 9, e103463, 2014.
51. Kowalski, P., Surowiak, P., Lage, H., Reversal of different drug-resistant phenotypes by an autocatalytic multitarget multiribozyme directed against the transcripts of the ABC transporters MDR1/P-gp, MRP2, and BCRP. *Mol. Ther.*, 11, 508–522, 2005.
52. Lo, Y.L. and Liu, Y., Reversing multi-drug resistance in Caco-2 by silencing MDR1, MRP1, MRP2, and BCL-2/BCL-xL using liposomal antisense oligonucleotides. *PLoS One*, 9, e90180, 2014.
53. Lo, Y.L., Liu, Y., Tsai, J.C., Overcoming multi-drug resistance using liposomal epirubicin and antisense oligonucleotides targeting pump and nonpump resistances *in vitro* and *in vivo*. *Biomed. Pharmacother.*, 67, 261–267, 2013.

54. Palmeira, A., Sousa, E., Vasconcelos, M.H., Pinto, M.M., Three decades of P-gp inhibitors: Skimming through several generations and scaffolds. *Curr. Med. Chem.*, 19, 1946–2025, 2012.
55. Li, X.Q., Wang, L., Lei, Y., Hu, T., Zhang, F.L., Cho, C.H., To, K.K., Reversal of P-gp and BCRP-mediated MDR by tariquidar derivatives. *Eur. J. Med. Chem.*, 101, 560–572, 2015.
56. Wu, C.P., Calcagno, A.M., Ambudkar, S.V., Reversal of ABC drug transporter-mediated multi-drug resistance in cancer cells: Evaluation of current strategies. *Curr. Mol. Pharmacol.*, 1, 93–105, 2008.
57. Crowley, E., McDevitt, C.A., Callaghan, R., Generating inhibitors of P-glycoprotein: Where to, now? *Methods Mol. Biol.*, 596, 405–432, 2010.
58. Benson, A.B. 3rd, Trump, D.L., Koeller, J.M., Egorin, M.I., Olman, E.A., Witte, R.S., Davis, T.E., Tormey, D.C., Phase I study of vinblastine and verapamil given by concurrent iv infusion. *Cancer Treat. Rep.*, 69, 795–799, 1985.
59. Yahanda, A.M., Alder, K.M., Fisher, G.A., Brophy, N.A., Halsey, J., Hardy, R.I., Gosland, M.P., Lum, B.L., Sikic, B.I., Phase I trial of etoposide with cyclosporine as a modulator of multi-drug resistance. *J. Clin. Oncol.*, 10, 1624–1634, 1992.
60. Warner, E., Hedley, D., Andrulis, I., Myers, R., Trudeau, M., Warr, D., Pritchard, K.I., Blackstein, M., Goss, P.E., Franssen, E. *et al.*, Phase II study of dexverapamil plus anthracycline in patients with metastatic breast cancer who have progressed on the same anthracycline regimen. *Clin. Cancer Res.*, 4, 1451–1457, 1998.
61. van der Holt, B., Löwenberg, B., Burnett, A.K., Knauf, W.U., Shepherd, J., Piccaluga, P.P., Ossenkoppele, G.J., Verhoef, G.E., Ferrant, A., Crump, M. *et al.*, The value of the MDR1 reversal agent PSC-833 in addition to daunorubicin and cytarabine in the treatment of elderly patients with previously untreated acute myeloid leukemia (AML), in relation to MDR1 status at diagnosis. *Blood*, 106, 2646–2654, 2005.
62. Pusztai, L., Wagner, P., Ibrahim, N., Rivera, E., Theriault, R., Booser, D., Symmans, F.W., Wong, F., Blumenschein, G., Fleming, D.R. *et al.*, Phase II study of tariquidar, a selective P-glycoprotein inhibitor, in patients with chemotherapy-resistant, advanced breast carcinoma. *Cancer*, 104, 682–691, 2005.
63. Zhang, W., Han, Y., Lim, S.L., Lim, L.Y., Dietary regulation of P-gp function and expression. *Expert Opin. Drug Metab. Toxicol.*, 5, 789–801, 2009.
64. Wu, C.P., Ohnuma, S., Ambudkar, S.V., Discovering natural product modulators to overcome multi-drug resistance in cancer chemotherapy. *Curr. Pharm. Biotechnol.*, 12, 609–620, 2011.
65. Li, Y., Revalde, J.L., Reid, G., Paxton, J.W., Interactions of dietary phytochemicals with ABC transporters: Possible implications for drug disposition and multi-drug resistance in cancer. *Drug Metab. Rev.*, 42, 590–611, 2010.

66. Hu, T., To, K.K., Wang, L., Zhang, L., Lu, L., Shen, J., Chan, R.L., Li, M., Yeung, J.H., Cho, C.H., Reversal of P-glycoprotein (P-gp) mediated multidrug resistance in colon cancer cells by cryptotanshinone and dihydrotanshinone of Salvia miltiorrhiza. *Phytomedicine*, 21, 1264–1272, 2014.
67. Zhang, Y., Zhang, Y.K., Wang, Y.J., Vispute, S.G., Jain, S., Chen, Y., Li, J., Youssef, D.T., El Sayed, K.A., Chen, Z.S., Esters of the marine-derived triterpene sipholenol A reverse P-GP-mediated drug resistance. *Mar. Drugs*, 13, 2267–2286, 2015.
68. Neerati, P., Sudhakar, Y.A., Kanwar, J.R., Curcumin regulates colon cancer by inhibiting p-glycoprotein in *in-situ* cancerous colon perfusion rat model. *J. Cancer Sci. Ther.*, 5, 313–319, 2013.
69. Nabekura, T., Overcoming multi-drug resistance in human cancer cells by natural compounds. *Toxins (Basel)*, 2, 1207–1224, 2010.
70. Lewis, A.D., Forrester, L.M., Hayes, J.D., Wareing, C.J., Carmichael, J., Harris, A.L., Mooghen, M., Wolf, C.R., Glutathione S-transferase isoenzymes in human tumours and tumour derived cell lines. *Br. J. Cancer*, 60, 327–331, 1989.
71. Hao, X.Y., Widersten, M., Ridderström, M., Hellman, U., Mannervik, B., Co-variation of glutathione transferase expression and cytostatic drug resistance in HeLa cells: Establishment of class Mu glutathione transferase M3-3 as the dominating isoenzyme. *Biochem. J.*, 297, Pt 1, 59–67, 1994.
72. Drake, F.H., Zimmerman, J.P., McCabe, F.L., Bartus, H.F., Per, S.R., Sullivan, D.M., Ross, W.E., Mattern, M.R., Johnson, R.K., Crooke, S.T., Purification of topoisomerase II from amsacrine-resistant P388 leukemia cells. Evidence for two forms of the enzyme. *J. Biol. Chem.*, 262, 16739–16747, 1987.
73. Fernald, K. and Kurokawa, M., Evading apoptosis in cancer. *Trends Cell Biol.*, 23, 620–633, 2013.
74. Reed, J.C., Regulation of apoptosis by bcl-2 family proteins and its role in cancer and chemoresistance. *Curr. Opin. Oncol.*, 7, 541–546, 1995.
75. Lowe, S.W., Schmitt, E.M., Smith, S.W., Osborne, B.A., Jacks, T., p53 is required for radiation-induced apoptosis in mouse thymocytes. *Nature*, 362, 847–849, 1993.
76. Tóthová, E., Fricova, M., Stecová, N., Kafková, A., Elbertová, A., High expression of bcl-2 protein in acute myeloid leukemia cells is associated with poor response to chemotherapy. *Neoplasma*, 49, 141–144, 2002.
77. Vacchelli, E., Senovilla, L., Eggermont, A., Fridman, W.H., Galon, J., Zitvogel, L., Kroemer, G., Galluzzi, L., Trial watch: Chemotherapy with immunogenic cell death inducers. *Oncoimmunology*, 2, e23510, 2013.
78. Zimmermann, K.C., Bonzon, C., Green, D.R., The machinery of programmed cell death. *Pharmacol. Ther.*, 92, 57–70, 2001.
79. Elmore, S., Apoptosis: A review of programmed cell death. *Toxicol. Pathol.*, **35**, 495–516, 2007.
80. Solary, E., Dubrez, L., Eymin, B., The role of apoptosis in the pathogenesis and treatment of diseases. *Eur. Respir. J.*, 9, 1293–1305, 1996.

81. Reed, J.C., Dysregulation of apoptosis in cancer. *J. Clin. Oncol.*, 17, 2941–2953, 1999.
82. Maiuri, M.C., Zalckvar, E., Kimchi, A., Kroemer, G., Self-eating and self-killing: Crosstalk between autophagy and apoptosis. *Nat. Rev. Mol. Cell Biol.*, 8, 741–752, 2007.
83. Kondo, Y., Kanzawa, T., Sawaya, R., Kondo, S., The role of autophagy in cancer development and response to therapy. *Nat. Rev. Cancer*, 5, 726–734, 2005.
84. Martinet, W. and De Meyer, G.R., Autophagy in atherosclerosis: A cell survival and death phenomenon with therapeutic potential. *Circ. Res.*, 104, 304–317, 2009.
85. Jiang, P. and Mizushima, N., Autophagy and human diseases. *Cell Res.*, 24, 69–79, 2014.
86. Cheng, Y., Ren, X., Hait, W.N., Yang, J.M., Therapeutic targeting of autophagy in disease: Biology and pharmacology. *Pharmacol. Rev.*, 65, 1162–1197, 2013.
87. Mizushima, N., Autophagy: Process and function. *Genes Dev.*, 21, 2861–2873, 2007.
88. Chapman, R.S., Whetton, A.D., Chresta, C.M., Dive, C., Characterization of drug resistance mediated via the suppression of apoptosis by Abelson protein tyrosine kinase. *Mol. Pharmacol.*, 48, 334–343, 1995.
89. Chapman, R.S., Whetton, A.D., Dive, C., The suppression of drug-induced apoptosis by activation of v-ABL protein tyrosine kinase. *Cancer Res.*, 54, 5131–5137, 1994.
90. Fulda, S., Tumor resistance to apoptosis. *Int. J. Cancer*, 124, 511–515, 2009.
91. Hu, T., Wang, L., Zhang, L., Lu, L., Shen, J., Chan, R.L., Li, M., Wu, W.K., To, K.K., Cho, C.H., Sensitivity of apoptosis-resistant colon cancer cells to tanshinones is mediated by autophagic cell death and p53-independent cytotoxicity. *Phytomedicine*, 22, 536–544, 2015.
92. Zhang, L., Yu, J., Park, B.H., Kinzler, K.W., Vogelstein, B., Role of BAX in the apoptotic response to anticancer agents. *Science*, 290, 989–992, 2000.
93. Herbst, R.S., Review of epidermal growth factor receptor biology. *Int. J. Radiat. Oncol. Biol. Phys.*, 59, 21–26, 2004.
94. Jorissen, R.N., Walker, F., Pouliot, N., Garrett, T.P., Ward, C.W., Burgess, A.W., Epidermal growth factor receptor: Mechanisms of activation and signalling. *Exp. Cell Res.*, 284, 31–53, 2003.
95. Goler-Garon, V., Sladkevich, I., Assaraf, Y.G., Inhibition of the PI3K-Akt signaling pathway disrupts ABCG2-rich extracellular vesicles and overcomes multi-drug resistance in breast cancer cells. *Biochem. Pharmacol.*, 83, 1340–8, 2012.
96. Stewart, C.F., Tagen, M., Schwartzberg, L.S., Blakely, L.J., Tauer, K.W., Smiley, L.M., Phase I dosage finding and pharmacokinetic study of intravenous Topotecan and oral Erlotinib in adults with refractory solid tumors. *Cancer Chemother. Pharmacol.*, 73, 561–8, 2014.

97. Bendell, J.C., Jones, S.F., Hart, L., Spigel, D.R., Lane, C.M., Earwood, C., Infante, J.R., Barton, J., Burris, H.A., A phase Ib study of linsitinib (OSI-906), a dual inhibitor of IGF-1R and IR tyrosine kinase, in combination with everolimus as treatment for patients with refractory metastatic colorectal cancer. *Investig. New Drugs*, 33, 187–93, 2015.
98. Tiwari, A.K., Sodani, K., Dai, C.L., Ashby Jr., C.R., Chen, Z.S., Revisiting the ABCs of multi-drug resistance in cancer chemotherapy. *Curr. Pharm. Biotechnol.*, 12, 570–94, 2011.
99. Chai, S., To, K.K., Lin, G., Circumvention of multi-drug resistance of cancer cells by Chinese herbal medicines. *Chin. Med.*, 5, 26, 2010.
100. Wang, Z., Xie, C., Huang, Y., Lam, C.W., Chow, M.S., Overcoming chemotherapy resistance with herbal medicines: Past, present and future perspectives. *Phytochem. Rev.*, 13, 323–37, 2014.
101. Ye, Q., Liu, K., Shen, Q., Li, Q., Hao, J., Han, F., Jiang, R.W., Reversal of multidrug resistance in cancer by multifunctional flavonoids. *Front. Oncol.*, 9, 487, 2019.
102. Alvarez, A.I., Real, R., Perez, M., Mendoza, G., Prieto, J.G., Merino, G., Modulation of the activity of ABC transporters (P-glycoprotein, MRP2, BCRP) by flavonoids and drug response. *J. Pharm. Sci.*, 99, 598–617, 2010.
103. Leslie, E.M., Mao, Q., Oleschuk, C.J., Deeley, R.G., Cole, S.P., Modulation of multi-drug resistance protein 1 (MRP1/ABCC1) transport and atpase activities by interaction with dietary flavonoids. *Mol. Pharmacol.*, 59, 1171–80, 2001.
104. Cooray, H.C., Janvilisri, T., van Veen, H.W., Hladky, S.B., Barrand, M.A., Interaction of the breast cancer resistance protein with plant polyphenols. *Biochem. Biophys. Res. Commun.*, 317, 269–75, 2004.
105. Lee, G., Joung, J.Y., Cho, J.H., Son, C.G., Lee, N., Overcoming p-glycoprotein-mediated multi-drug resistance in colorectal cancer: Potential reversal agents among herbal medicines. *Evid. Based Complement. Alternat. Med.*, 3412074, 3–4, 2018.
106. Li, H., Krstin, S., Wang, S., Wink, M., Capsaicin and piperine can overcome multi-drug resistance in cancer cells to doxorubicin. *Molecules*, 23, 3, 1–2, 2018. https://doi.org/10.3390/molecules23030557. pii: E557.
107. Li, H., Krstin, S., Wink, M., Modulation of multi-drug resistant in cancer cells by EGCG, tannic acid and curcumin. *Phytomedicine*, 50, 213–22, 2018.
108. Zhou, J.X. and Wink, M., Reversal of multi-drug resistance in human colon cancer and human leukemia cells by three plant extracts and their major secondary metabolites. *Medicines (Basel)*, 5, 4, 123, 2018. https://doi.org/10.3390/ medicines5040123. pii: E123.
109. Syed, S.B., Arya, H., Fu, I.H., Yeh, T.K., Periyasamy, L., Hsieh, H.P., Coumar, M.S., Targeting P-glycoprotein: Investigation of piperine analogs for overcoming, drug resistance in cancer. *Sci. Rep.*, 7, 7972, 2017.
110. Huang, L., Zhang, S., Zhou, J., Li, X., Effect of resveratrol on drug resistance in colon cancer chemotherapy. *RSC Adv.*, 9, 2572–80, 2019.

111. Guo, P., Wang, J., Gao, W., Liu, X., Wu, S., Wang, B., Xu, L., Li, Y., Salvianolic acid B reverses multi-drug resistance in nude mice bearing human colon cancer stem cells. *Mol. Med. Rep.*, 18, 1323–34, 2018.
112. Bhardwaj, M., Cho, H.J., Paul, S., Jakhar, R., Khan, I., Lee, S.J., Kim, B.Y., Krishnan, M., Khaket, T.P., Lee, H.G., Kang, S.C., Vitexin induces apoptosis by suppressing autophagy in multi-drug resistant colorectal cancer cells. *Oncotarget*, 9, 3278–91, 2018.
113. Forester, S.C. and Waterhouse, A.L., Metabolites are key to understanding health effects of wine polyphenols. *J. Nutr.*, 139, S1824–31, 2009.
114. Bohn, T., McDougall, G.J., Alegria, A., Alminger, M., Arrigoni, E., Aura, A.M., Brito, C., Cilla, A., El, S.N., Karakaya, S., Martinez-Cuesta, M.C., Santos, C.N., Mind the gap-deficits in our knowledge of aspects impacting the bioavailability of phytochemicals and their metabolites—A position paper focusing on carotenoids and polyphenols. *Mol. Nutr. Food Res.*, 59, 1307–23, 2015.
115. To, K.K., MicroRNA: A prognostic biomarker and a possible druggable target for circumventing multi-drug resistance in cancer chemotherapy. *J. Biomed. Sci.*, 20, 99, 2013.
116. To, K.K., Robey, R.W., Knutsen, T., Zhan, Z., Ried, T., Bates, S.E., Escape from hsa-miR-519c enables drug resistant cells to maintain high expression of ABCG2. *Mol. Cancer Ther.*, 9, 2959–68, 2009.
117. Peng, S.S., Chen, C.Y., Xy, N., Shyu, A.B., RNA stabilization by the AU-rich element binding protein, HuR, an ELAV protein. *EMBO J.*, 17, 3461–70, 1998.
118. To, K.K., Leung, W.W., Ng, S.S., Exploiting a novel miR-519c-HuR-ABCG2 regulatory pathway to overcome chemoresistance in colorectal cancer. *Exp. Cell Res.*, 338, 222–31, 2015.
119. Jacobson, K.A., Balasubramanian, R., Deflorian, F., Gao, Z.G., G protein-coupled adenosine (P1) and P2Y receptors: Ligand design and receptor interactions. *Puringergic Signal.*, 8, 419–36, 2012.
120. Shabbir, M., Ryten, M., Thompson, C., Mikhailidis, D., Burnstock, G., Purinergic receptor-mediated effects of ATP in high-grade bladder cancer. *BJU Int.*, 101, 106–12, 2008.
121. Agteresch, H.J., Burgers, S.A., van der Gaast, A., Wilson, J.H., Dagnelie, P.C., Randomized clinical trial of adenosine 50 -triphosphate on tumor growth and survival in advanced lung cancer patients. *Anticancer Drugs*, 14, 639–44, 2003.
122. Swennen, E.L., Ummels, V., Buss, I., Jaehde, U., Bast, A., Dagnelie, P.C., ATP sensitizes H460 lung carcinoma cells to cisplatin-induced apoptosis. *Chem. Bio Interact.*, 184, 338–45, 2010.
123. Buzzi, N., Boland, R., Russo de Boland, A., Signal transduction pathways associated with ATP-induced proliferation of colon adenocarcinoma cells. *Biochim. Biophys. Acta*, 2010, 946–55, 1800.

124. Vinette, V., Placet, M., Arguin, G., Gendron, F.P., Multi-drug resistance-associated protein 2 expression is upregulated by adenosine 5'-triphosphate in colorectal cancer cells and enhances their survival to chemotherapeutic drugs. *PLoS One*, 10, 4–6, 2015.
125. Beck, W.T., Grogan, T.M., Willman, C.L., Cordon-Cardo, C., Parham, D.M., Kuttesch, J.F. *et al.*, Methods to detect P-glycoprotein-associated multi-drug resistance in patients' tumors: Consensus recommendations. *Cancer Res.*, 56, 3010–20, 1996.
126. Agrawal, M. *et al.*, Increased 99mTc-sestamibi accumulation in normal liver and drug-resistant tumors after the administration of the glycoprotein inhibitor, XR9576. *Clin. Cancer Res.*, 9, 650–6, 2003.
127. Sargent, D.J., Marsoni, S., Monges, G., Thibodeau, S.N., Labianca, R., Hamilton, S.R. *et al.*, Defective mismatch repair as a predictive marker for lack of efficacy of fluorouracil-based adjuvant therapy in colon cancer. *J. Clin. Oncol.*, 28, 3219–26, 2010.
128. Al-Hajeili, M., Shields, A.F., Hwang, J.J., Wadlow, R.C., Marshall, J.L., Molecular testing to optimize and personalize decision making in the management of colorectal cancer. *Oncol. (Williston Park, NY)*, 31, 301–12, 2017.

7

Epithelial to Mesenchymal Transition (EMT): Major Contribution to Cancer Drug Therapy Resistance

Rishabha Malviya*, Arun Kumar Singh and Deepika Yadav

Abstract

Using drug-targeting tactics, significant clinical gains have been made in the treatment of cancer patients during the last decade. However, medication resistance remains a critical issue in many cancer treatments. The tumor microenvironment and epithelial-mesenchymal plasticity (EMP) have been cited as factors in the difficulty of treating several cancer types. Epithelial-to-mesenchymal transition (EMT) has also been linked to treatment resistance in a number of preclinical models, while clinical trials and clinical samples have not confirmed this. The effect of intermediate epithelial/mesenchymal (E/M) states and their relationship to the microenvironment on treatment resistance will be covered in this chapter. The author also discuss the potential uses of pharmacogenomics and bioinformatics in determining how the EMT affects drug resistance biologically and in the development of more effective therapeutic approaches.

Keywords: Epithelial plasticity, therapy resistance, tumor microenvironment, cancer, EMT, tumor resistance

7.1 Introduction

Overcoming therapeutic resistance is one of the most pressing issues in oncology right now because it is so difficult to treat cancer patients who have developed immunity to their treatments. Since metastasis is the leading cause of mortality in patients with human carcinomas, it is crucial to find methods of treating individuals who have developed resistance to treatment

**Corresponding author*: rishabhamalviya19@gmail.com

Rishabha Malviya, Arun Kumar Singh and Deepika Yadav. Multi-Drug Resistance in Cancer: Mechanism and Treatment Strategies, (131–154) © 2023 Scrivener Publishing LLC

[1–4]. Cancer cells can develop resistance to a wide variety of therapies, including the more well-known innate and acquired forms of resistance as well as chemotherapy, radiation therapy, immunological therapies, and others. Drug resistance is mostly caused by molecular alterations, such as altered expression of anti-apoptotic proteins, increased efflux caused by overexpressed MDR efflux transporters, and decreased absorption caused by altered influx transporters [5]. However, the molecular mechanisms that result in treatment resistance are still incompletely understood.

Epithelial-to-mesenchymal transition (EMT) has been connected to the emergence of drug resistance in recent studies. EMT is a biological process that transforms polarized, immobile epithelial cells into mesenchymal, motile cells by rearranging the actin cytoskeleton, removing apicobasal polarity, creating cell-cell connections, and entering the extracellular matrix as a single cell [6]. The main cause of treatment resistance, both to conventional treatments and to small-molecule targeted inhibitors, is the EMT phenotype, which is connected to the growth and spread of tumors.

Tumor cell lines have been used to show that EMT contributes to resistance to radiotherapy and chemotherapy. There is a lack of *in vivo* data due, in large part, to a lack of appropriate *in vivo* models and a lack of human samples for analysis [7]. In contrast, carcinomas display a heterogeneous E/M phenotypic state, which leads to the presence of distinct subpopulations and an overall increase in tumor plasticity [8]. However, evidence from pharmacogenomics studies suggests that intermediate E/M states are relevant in predicting a patient's response to anticancer therapies [9]. The significance of individualized cancer treatment has been highlighted by the discovery of a critical connection between EMT and the tumor microenvironment.

There is now no need for more study on the topic since there is so much high-quality, newly published literature on the topic of the tumor microenvironment and EMT in MDR. In this article, the investigator explored whether or not the setting influences the success of EMT treatment. Possible bioinformatic and pharmaceutical strategies to overcome therapy resistance will also be analyzed from a future perspective [10–13].

7.2 EMT and Tumor Resistance: *In Vitro, In Vivo,* and Clinical Trials

Through a series of molecular and cellular changes known as the EMT program, cancerous epithelial tumor cells lose their epithelial identity and take on a mesenchymal phenotype. The plasticity and reversibility of EMT are exemplified by the mesenchymal-to-epithelial transition (MET), a process by which mesenchymal cells acquire an epithelial phenotype. High epithelial-mesenchymal plasticity leads to the E/M hybrid phenotypes that are characteristic of tumors (EMP). Epithelial-mesenchymal plasticity is governed by transcriptional, post-transcriptional, and post-translational pathways that are highly controlled and have important clinical consequences [13–15]. N-cadherin, Vimentin, and Fibronectin are epithelial markers, whereas cytokeratins and claudins are mesenchymal markers. Twist, Zeb1, and Zeb2 are Snail/Slug family members and crucial EMT proteins. Both transcriptional regulators, including the miR-200 family and RNA-binding proteins, and post-translational regulators, such as phosphatases, control the degradation of E-cadherin [16].

Numerous studies have examined EMT's impact on cancer metastasis. But there are canonical works that dispute the necessity of EMT in this context. Still, there is mounting proof linking EMT to resistance to treatment. EMT and cancer stemness have been studied concerning treatment resistance in the current scientific literature [17]. Drug resistance is often connected with EMT for the following reasons: reduced cell growth, decreased drug efflux, and avoidance of apoptotic signaling pathways. Treatment resistance due to EMT is mostly attributable to changes in the mRNA expression of molecules involved in immunosuppression and immunoevasion. The effect of EMT on drug resistance has been shown in a number of *in vitro* and animal models, despite the fact that the precise molecular mechanism by which EMT has this effect is poorly understood [18]. Research into EMT's effects has been conducted *in vitro*, *in vivo*, and in human tissue. Reportedly, transcriptional or post-translational regulators of EMT are linked to cancer drug resistance. In this chapter, the focus has been on the most recent research on EMT in several mouse models of cancer.

Studies using transgenic mice as *in vivo* models have produced some of the most controversial results in this area [19]. Triple transgenic mice with breast cancer that overexpressed miR-200a regained sensitivity to cyclophosphamide and had their EMT-TFs Zeb1 and Zeb2 silenced. Genomically modified animal models of pancreatic ductal cancer revealed increased susceptibility to gemcitabine after Snail and Twist TF deletion. In both studies, researchers looked for evidence that EMT contributed to cancer metastasis, but they came up empty [20–22]. These two *in vivo* preclinical models illustrate the potential value of coupling EMT inhibition with chemotherapy in the treatment of cancer by providing considerable evidence for EMT's participation as a driving factor behind drug resistance.

The two studies using transgenic mice are important, but *in vitro* research, xenograft tumors in athymic mice, and clinical specimens provide the best evidence between EMT and chemoresistance. Some of the strongest evidence connecting EMT and therapy resistance can be found in lung cancer [23–25]. In EGFR mutant NSCLC, inhibiting FGFR has been shown to be an efficient method of overcoming the resistance brought on by EMT. In EGFR-mutant NSCLC, resistance to gefitinib and EMT are acquired via the epigenetic silencing of miR-483-3p, while none of these processes takes place in non-EGFR-mutant NSCLC. Numerous studies have shown a link between EMT-TFs and medication resistance. For instance, overexpression of Snail and Slug has been linked to treatment resistance in lung cancer cell lines with EGFR mutations. "It has also been shown that PAX6 regulates Zeb2 expression, causing EMT and cisplatin resistance. Epithelial-mesenchymal transition-associated gene AXL amplification has been linked to acquired resistance to the EGFR-TKI osimertinib [26, 27]. A number of mechanisms, including cell stem features, inhibition of the proapoptotic protein Bcl-2-like protein 11, and chromatin remodeling mediated by EMT-TFs, have been postulated to explain this therapeutic resistance. Additionally, MET-driven EMT can initiate chemoresistance. Cell lines derived from cisplatin-resistant NSCLC tumors showed overexpression of MET, as well as elevated levels of N-cadherin, Vimentin, Zeb1, and Snail expression and reduced levels of E-cadherin expression. After MET was downregulated by mir-206, NSCLC cells reverted EMT and became susceptible to cisplatin.EMT and tumor resistance are represented in Figure 7.1.

Twist, Snail, and FOXC2 are three TFs whose overexpression increases the activity of ABC transporter promoters and raises the possibility that EMT inducers are new regulators of ABC transporters in breast cancer [28]. This has led researchers to consider EMT-TFs as a novel strategy for combating metastasis and the treatment resistance it breeds. Epithelial-to-mesenchymal transition (E/M) phenotype breast cancer cells have been shown to acquire drug resistance and metastasize more effectively than fully mesenchymal breast cancer cells. It has been suggested that Zeb1 downregulates ITGB4 expression in mesenchymal-like triple-negative breast cancer cells as a possible biological mechanism for ITGB4-mediated resistance. That's because Tap63 upregulates ITGB4 expression [29]. Two more significant examples of how EMT-TFs contribute to drug resistance are the overexpression of Twist or the inhibition of E-cadherin activation in healthy and transformed human mammary epithelial cells. Snail transforms the sensitive basal-like MDA-MB-231 breast cancer cells into drug-resistant tumor cells. However, paclitaxel may destroy breast cancer cells that have a

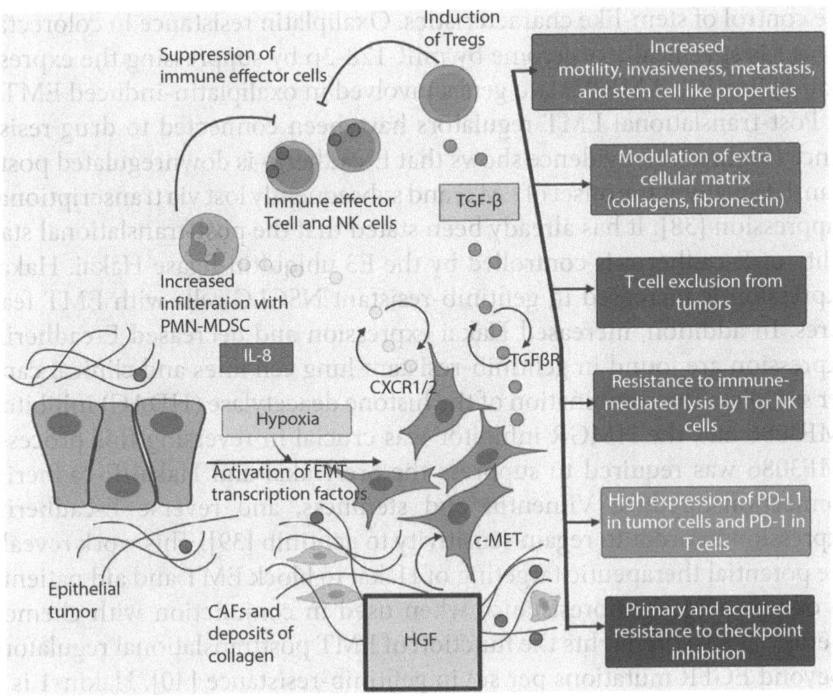

Figure 7.1 Schematic representation of EMT and tumor resistance.

mesenchymal phenotype. This study contributes to the increasing body of evidence suggesting cancer cells undergoing EMT are more susceptible to endoplasmic reticulum stress because inducing EMT increases PERK-eIF2 and makes cells more susceptible to drugs that impair endoplasmic reticulum function [30–35]. EMT and endocrine therapy resistance in luminal breast cancer have been related causally using *in vitro* and xenograft models. In breast cancer cell lines that generate fusion proteins derived from the oestrogen receptor alpha gene, overexpression of Snail and downregulation of E-cadherin promote estrogen-independent activation of EMT (ESR1). Additionally, EMT has been linked to therapeutic resistance in prostate and ovarian cancers. In androgen-sensitive tumors, antiandrogen-mediated EMT-MET may circumvent cabazitaxel resistance, even though patients with metastatic castration-resistant prostate cancer typically acquire therapeutic resistance to taxane chemotherapy and antiandrogens. However, prostate cancer cells and the xenograft mouse model acquire resistance to radiation thanks to the EMT-inducing protein Lysyl oxidase-like 2 (LOXL2) [36, 37]. The EMT-TFs Snail and Slug support chemoresistance and radioresistance in ovarian cancer via p53-driven apoptosis and the control of stem-like characteristics. Oxaliplatin resistance in colorectal cancer is specifically overcome by miR-128-3p by suppressing the expression of Bmi1 and MRP5, two genes involved in oxaliplatin-induced EMT.

Post-translational EMT regulators have been connected to drug resistance (Figure 7.1). Evidence shows that E-cadherin is downregulated post-translationally at the onset of EMT, and subsequently lost via transcriptional suppression [38]. It has already been stated that the post-translational stability of E-cadherin is controlled by the E3 ubiquitin-ligase Hakai. Hakai expression is increased in gefitinib-resistant NSCLC cells with EMT features. In addition, increased Hakai expression and decreased E-cadherin expression are found in gefitinib-resistant lung cell lines and clinical cancer samples. The combination of the histone deacetylase (HDAC) inhibitor JMF3086 and the HMGR inhibitor was crucial in reversing this process. JMF3086 was required to suppress the Src/Hakai and Hakai/E-cadherin connections, reduce Vimentin and stemness, and reverse E-cadherin expression in order to regain sensitivity to gefitinib [39]. This work reveals the potential therapeutic targeting of Hakai to block EMT and aid patients in overcoming chemoresistance when used in conjunction with chemotherapy. It also highlights the function of EMT posttranslational regulators (beyond EGFR mutations per se) in gefitinib-resistance [40]. Hakin-1 is a rare selective small-molecule inhibitor of Hakai, according to the current study, which raises the possibility that it might be a useful therapeutic agent for the prevention of EMT. Hakai's mode of action suggests it may be effective against numerous forms of cancer, including lung and gastrointestinal. In this chapter, a potentially essential post-translational mechanism in colorectal cancer that may alter therapy resistance is reported. The F-Box E3 ubiquitin ligase FBXW7 degrades the transcription factor Zeb2 as a result of GSK3 phosphorylation in intestinal stem cells [41]. Increasing chemoresistance, EMT, and metastasis in mice and human colorectal cancer cell lines is the Zeb2/FBXW7 axis. The ubiquitin-proteasome system may have a role in both breast and pancreatic cancer, according to recent research. The Snail protein is stabilized by the deubiquitinase USP27X, which is active during TGF-induced EMT. The fact that Snail may be degraded and cisplatin can be more effective when USP27X is absent suggests a need for novel therapeutic strategies to overcome chemoresistance.

7.3 Tumor Microenvironment Regulates EMT

The microenvironment of a solid tumor refers to the specific community of tumor cells (TME). In addition to tumor cells, the tumor microenvironment

(TME) contains a wide variety of other cell types. This group of cells includes myeloid cells, lymphoid cells (such as T cells, B cells, and NK cells), endothelial cells, and fibroblasts (such as macrophages, granulocytes, and lymphocytes) [42]. The extracellular matrix (ECM), a massive network of macromolecules, predominates in the acellular component of the TME. The TME also includes the soluble compounds secreted by the cells that make up the microenvironment, such as enzymes, cytokines, chemokines, and antibodies [43–45]. In most solid tumors, hypoxia is a feature of the tumor microenvironment (TME), and the TME metabolome frequently differs from that of the normal organ. In addition, the tumor microenvironment of treated tumor carriers may contain drugs (TME). Tumor cells and their molecular products interact with host cells and chemicals to form the tumor microenvironment (TME). Tumor-host interactions can cause metastasis and therapeutic resistance by reprogramming both the tumor and the host phenotype.

Cancer cells are able to thrive, multiply, and metastasize not only due to their own intrinsic mechanisms but also through interaction with neighboring cells and the extracellular matrix. There is a complicated chain of events that cancer cells must go through as they invade and colonize new organs [46]. Tumor-derived and TME-derived factors work together to regulate each stage of the metastatic cascade. The ability of tumor cells to invade neighboring tissues is one of the earliest events in the process of metastasis, and it is achieved through the activation of the EMT program. The cells then undergo a process called metastasis in which they start to spread to different organs [47]. The EMT program is set in motion by paracrine signals from the tumor microenvironment (TME) released by non-tumorigenic cells such as fibroblasts, macrophages, or immunocytes that are either present in the tumor or invading the tumor [48]. The EMT-driving molecular program, which operates via a network of interconnected and mutually reinforcing signaling pathways, uses the microenvironment as its activating environment. These include cytokines, growth factors, integrins, microRNAs, proteins of the extracellular matrix (ECM), and TGF-s. Many transcription factors involved in the epithelial-mesenchymal transition are upregulated by the signaling pathways described here, some of which may be redundant (EMT) [49, 50].

Factors involved in EMT coordinate the processes by which cells alter their shape, increase their motility, reprogram the extracellular matrix, and decrease their tight junctions. Some solid tumors include preexisting tumor subpopulations with characteristics ranging from totally epithelial to entirely mesenchymal [51]. This is because the EMT process has distinct intermediate stages. It is possible that the host cells in the

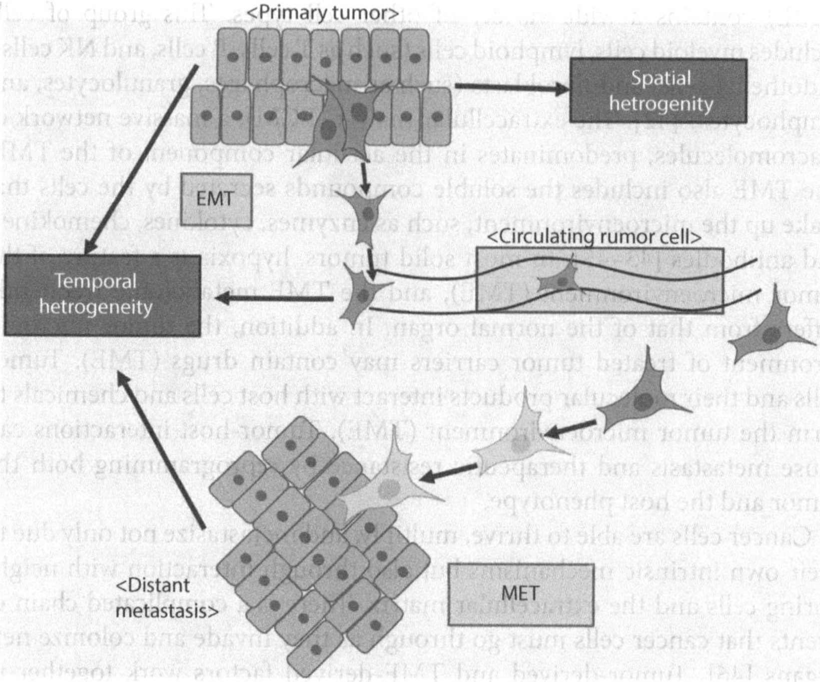

Figure 7.2 Potential therapeutic target for reversing treatment resistance: the microenvironmental drivers of the EMT.

microenvironment, which are linked to various tumor subpopulations, also display some degree of diversity. Remember that mesenchymal-tumor cells are produced as a result of the EMT process and that these cells have varying effects on the microenvironmental cells, which may in turn affect tumor growth and treatment resistance. Several key elements of the local environment that can trigger EMT are discussed below (Figure 7.2).

7.3.1 Hypoxia

An EMT-inducing hypoxic microenvironment is present in nearly all solid tumors. Hypoxia-Inducible Factors (HIFs), a family of transcriptional regulators involved in extracellular matrix (ECM) maintenance and repair, cell survival and proliferation, metabolism, inflammation, and angiogenesis, promote tumor development. Both the EMT process and the development of drug resistance include high-impact genes (HIFs) [52]. Multiple transcription factors that play a role in generating EMT have their expression and activity boosted by HIF-1. Such elements consist of Twist,

Zeb1, and Snail. EMT might be sent in response to any of these potential triggers. Such chemicals prevent tumor cells from producing epithelial-specific proteins like E-cadherin, giving them a more mesenchymal look. HIF-1's effect may be mediated by its interactions with other factors. Some of the most powerful inducers of EMT are members of the TGF family, with which HIF-1 interacts (the significance of the TGF-family in EMT is addressed in further detail below). These two partners work together to aid EMT [53–55].

7.3.2 The Extracellular Matrix

The extracellular matrix (ECM) is a component of the tissue microenvironment (TME) that offers the cells in a given milieu both structural and biochemical support. The adhesion and communication between cells are facilitated. Integrins, collagen, glycoproteins, glycosaminoglycans, and enzymes are all examples of macromolecules that may be found in the extracellular matrix (ECM) [56]. Tzanakakis's study, by analyzing their interactions, provides a comprehensive overview of the ECM components that regulate EMT. Deregulated ECM remodeling has a major impact on tumor development and may be triggered by matricellular proteins, ROS, hypoxia, or proteases. Alterations in proteoglycan expression, collagen interactome reorganization, proteolytic destruction of macromolecules, and integrin activation are all possible during ECM remodeling. The EMT process is triggered by the abovementioned changes to the structure and function of the extracellular matrix.

7.3.3 The Inflammatory and Immune Microenvironment

Immunocytes, inflammatory cells, and their chemical products both promote and inhibit tumor growth in the tumor microenvironment (TME) [57, 58]. To some extent, EMT may be initiated, driven, and maintained by the secretome of inflammatory cells. A tumor-associated macrophage is a macrophage that has made its way into a tumor (TAMs). By secreting the angiogenic cytokine VEGF and pro-inflammatory cytokines, these cells facilitate the spread of the tumor. By secreting pro-inflammatory cytokines such as TNF-, TGF-, IL-1, IL-6, CCL5, and CCL18, TAMs play a critical role in the initiation and maintenance of EMT. TAMs may begin EMT in a variety of ways. EMT is also thought to involve cells of the myeloid lineage, which includes granulocytes and myeloid-derived suppressor cells. Lymphocytes, such as regulatory T cells, that infiltrate tumors can trigger EMT by producing inflammatory and tumor-promoting cytokines [59].

Due to the interplay between the tumor and its microenvironment, NK cells with atypical phenotypes drive metastasis rather than suppress it. This is why the activation of EMT is employed in the promotion of metastasis [60]. Infiltrating NK cells promote tumor growth and metastasis by activating matrix metalloproteinases and promoting the production of IL-6 and other pro-inflammatory cytokines. During EMT, cancer cells may take on immunosuppressive characteristics or change their immunogenicity, allowing them to evade anti-tumor immune responses or causing the emergence of novel tumor-associated epitopes.

7.3.4 EMT Microenvironment: Medication Resistance

The tumor microenvironment controls the EMT, which contributes to resistance to therapy. EMT-related treatment resistance may be regulated by signals from the tumor stroma, such as growth factors or cytokines, according to a number of studies [61]. Many components of the extracellular matrix, such as hyaluronan and transforming growth factor-1, are secreted by CAFs. This article demonstrates how the properties of hyaluronan in cancer resistance may make cells more sensitive to contact inhibition and cell cycle arrest using naked rat mole fibroblasts as a model system [62–65]. More motile than CAFs that synthesize more transforming growth factor beta 1 are CAFs that sustain high levels of hyaluronan production through autocrine processes. However, TGF-1 did increase invasion and EMT markers without increasing motility, indicating separate mechanisms are at work in carcinoma progression. Therefore, tumor stromal cell-secreted TGF-drives a common gene program among poor-prognosis colorectal cancer subtypes, suggesting a connection to treatment resistance [66]. Antigen-presenting cells' production of IL-6 encourages TGF-induced EMT in non-small lung cancer cells (NSCLS). The researcher assumed that IL-6 aids in the production of a paracrine loop that intercommunicated CAFs and NSCLS, resulting in chemoresistance, since cisplatin treatment elevated TGF-expression and conditioned media from cancer cells stimulated fibroblasts. Inducing gemcitabine resistance, the IL6 cytokine oncostatin M (OSM) increased the expression of Zeb1, Snail (SNAI1), and OSM receptor in pancreatic ductal adenocarcinoma cells [67].

Hypoxia is related to treatment resistance and is prevalent in the microenvironment of solid tumors. Hypoxia activates the hypoxia-inducible gene procollagen-lysine 2-oxoglutarate 5-dioxygenase 2 in biliary tract cancer cells, and EMT is associated with gemcitabine resistance (PLOD2). The transcription factor HIF-1 has been linked to resistance to treatment. Evidence supporting the use of a pharmacologic modification of HIF-1 as a treatment method to overcome resistance to gemcitabine comes from the discovery of a correlation between EMT and HIF-1 activation in pancreatic cancer cells. Because they carry chemicals that affect tumor growth, exosomes are to blame for medication resistance. Exosomes secreted by tumor cells may help the tumor microenvironment in promoting treatment resistance and EMT. EMT is a mechanism via which exosomal miR-155 is linked to resistance to both cisplatin and paclitaxel in gastric cancer cells [68].

Likewise noteworthy is the effect of the tumor's immune microenvironment on EMT and treatment resistance. Proteins called chemokines and cytokines are secreted by cancer cells to entice specific types of immune cells to aid in the fight against the tumor [69]. The epigenetic regulator Snail is thought to promote tumor-associated macrophage inflammation and resistance to anticancer therapy in a variety of malignancies, including lung cancer, by suppressing the expression of ubiquitin-specific protease 4 (USP4) [70]. Cancer patients now have immunotherapy as a potential treatment options thanks to recent promising results. Interfering with PD-1's interaction with PDL-1 or CTLA-4 has been proven to be a promising approach to treating cancer using immune inhibitors [71]. Further research is required to completely understand the molecular mechanism of immune escape, however evidence has arisen supporting EMT's function in immune escape, and the potential value of EMT markers has been outlined for immunological therapy selection. Recurrent cancer patients treated with the PD-L1 inhibitor nivulumab showed that their cancer stem cells (CTCs) co-expressed the EMT markers N-cadherin and Vimentin [72].

These findings provide credence to the concept that EMT and PDL-1 might be used to determine whether individuals are likely to have an inadequate response to immunotherapy. EMT has been connected to immunosuppression, which is associated with CD8+ tumor-infiltrating lymphocytes (TILs). In this case, the target of miR-200 is PD-L1 [73]. By down-regulating miR-200, Zeb1 decreases miR-200's ability to control PD-L1 on tumor cells, which in turn reduces CD8+ T-cell immunity. Patients whose tumors are driven by EMT activators had a better chance of benefiting from PD-L1 inhibitors, according to the results of this groundbreaking research. Another method with the potential for predicting treatment response and survival is the EMT transcriptional score. Based on the EMT-transcriptional score in different tumor types, patients with a luminal phenotype (more epithelial phenotype) cancer tend to have better responses to immunotherapy (mesenchymal phenotype) [74]. It is important to note that mesenchymal-like tumors are not intrinsically resistant to chemotherapy since they reacted differentially to therapeutic administration with or without paclitaxel, demonstrating a difference in phenotype between epithelial and mesenchymal-like ovarian malignancies. High EMT-score tumors, such as those found in the lung and the head and neck, tend to express immune expression indicators like PDL-1. The impact of the microenvironment on EMT and therapeutic resistance needs more investigation. Investigation of EMT-induced treatment resistance has to include, among other things, pharmacology and bioinformatics.

7.4 Drug Resistance and EMT Bioinformatics

7.4.1 Bioinformatics and Pharmacogenomics to Optimize Drugs and Targets and Identify Medication Resistance

Understanding clinically relevant phenotypic programming is essential for developing precisely targeted medicines, and future advances in bioinformatics will play a crucial role in this endeavor [75]. Bioinformatics and patient samples will help examine the biological effect of EMT depending on the transition dynamics as the role of EMT in medication resistance is not completely known. Numerous important studies have investigated EMT and its potential role in drug resistance using mathematical or computational methods. Example: Mathematical modeling using RACIPE has shown a favorable association between Twist1 and Vimentin and a substantial adverse relationship with E-cadherin [76]. Twist1 overexpression during EMT has been linked to an increase in genomic instability, which in turn has been linked to an increase in cellular diversity and resistance to chemotherapy. To recover lost gene expression from single-cell data, a recent computer method dubbed MAGIC (Markov affinity-based graph imputation of cells) was developed [77]. The stem-like characteristics of a significant fraction of cells in the E/M transitional stage are shown by MAGIC. It is interesting to note that drug resistance appears to be highest at a moderate activation level of the EMT-program in carcinoma cells. Foroutan *et al.* used a systematic bioinformatics approach to reveal that the TGF-driven EMT pathway is surprisingly devoid of mutations [78]. Low- and high-scoring cell lines also responded differently to a variety of standard cancer treatments. Tumor types with a high score included fewer mutations in the TGF pathway and had considerably poorer survival rates compared to data from The Cancer Genome Atlas' complete tumor collection [79]. To back up the idea of a drug-specific impact, the pan-drug investigation showed that TGF-induced EMT was not followed by systemic drug resistance.

Within the context of genome-wide studies, pharmacogenomics is a rapidly expanding field that studies how human gene products, or proteins, influence the response to medications and pharmacological treatments [80]. By integrating pharmacology and genetics, researchers in this emerging field hope to create personalized cancer therapies that are less toxic and more effective for individual patients. The specific molecular interaction of many drugs is frequently unclear and may vary widely across people, but it is generally understood that medications may function on a range of molecular targets within the body [81]. More accurate mapping of the molecular targets of each treatment needs extensive genomic and proteomic data linked to drug activity in human cells. This method of mapping drug-target interactions has been very helpful in the field of cancer genomics, enabling the testing of hundreds of anti-cancer drugs in a variety of human cancer cell lines. To better understand the biological basis for variations in treatment response, researchers should integrate genomic data with pharmacological activity [82]. For this reason, pharmacogenomics seeks to find particular genetic variables that influence reactivity or resistance in cancer patients to medications; this information might be significant for understanding the safety, toxicity, and effectiveness of therapies in individual patients or groups of patients. The CYP2D6 gene, which encodes a cytochrome P450 involved in the metabolism of 25% of all presently prescribed drugs, has been revealed to include a large number of genetic variations. An individual gene variant can have a major impact on how well a treatment works. Studies involving people with breast cancer have revealed that CYP2D6 allelic variants play a major role in determining tamoxifen's efficacy and safety. Erlotinib, gefetinib, and afatinib were used to treat malignancies, and pharmacogenomics research has been done to find reasons for resistance, such as the overexpression or amplification of other genes including MET and HER2 [83].

The field of pharmacogenomics holds promise for the correction of the all-too-common issue of insufficient medication response. Drug inefficiency, which is frequently linked to distinct individual variability, can be significantly influenced by the complexity of drug interactions (resulting from the existence of numerous drug targets, drug-drug cross-reactions, target-to-target interferences, etc.) and the impact of multiple environmental factors. There is a lot of data to support the idea that heritable factors (such as differences in drug targets, drug metabolizing enzymes, and/or drug transporters) have a role in drug resistance. The presence of multiple-drug resistance proteins, for instance, may be related to a patient's unique resistance level (MRPs). These proteins play a crucial role in the evolution of resistance to many different types of anticancer medicines, and they exhibit genetic polymorphisms that generate considerable inter-individual variation in expression and activity.

7.4.2 Drug Resistance: Hereditary or Acquired

Unfortunately, genetic and acquired resistance are major roadblocks to target-driven anticancer therapy (defined as secondary resistance) [84]. Resistance may develop amongst individuals with the same tumor type or even within a single tumor mass, indicating the phenotypic variety of cancer cells cohabiting with the mass. Since drug resistance tends to be genetic, the varying manifestations of cancer among individuals should come as no surprise. Second, intra-tumor heterogeneity in cancer is frequently linked to treatment resistance. Both types of drug resistance have been explained by recent advances in pharmaceutical genomics. Small-molecule tyrosine kinase inhibitor (TKI) resistance is often established and progresses at varying rates in different people. Genome-wide analyses have shown that resistant individuals possessed somatic point mutations in NTRK1, KDR, TGFBR2, and PTPN11, as well as copy number variations in CDK4, CDKN2B, and ERBB2z.

7.4.3 Therapies for EMT-Induced Medication Resistance

Since EMT plays a role in both cancer metastasis and treatment resistance, inhibiting it may be a valuable therapeutic strategy for treating cancer [85]. There is intriguing evidence linking drug resistance to epithelial or mesenchymal cell types, as was just mentioned. The investigator made hypothesis that focusing on these states by focusing on their regulators might be a strategy to overcome or slow down the course of sickness since there is now research, including the possibility that the specific condition of these two phenomena could be changeable (Brozovic, unpublished data) [86]. On the subject of therapeutic targets, small-molecule inhibitors of tumor plasticity, and natural compounds that may be used to combat cancer metastasis, several excellent reviews have been produced. There was also a look at the research done on drugs and chemicals that have been shown to inhibit EMT in the environment. DNA methylation, histone modifications, and other epigenetic mechanisms have been shown to regulate many EMT drivers, suggesting that they may be useful therapeutic targets for suppressing EMT. Transcription factors, environmental factors, signaling pathways, RNA-binding proteins, and microRNAs are only some of the mediators that control EMT. Drug-resistant EMT targets are widespread, supporting this theory [87–89]. Although it is impossible to provide an in-depth analysis of each target, this review will concentrate on those that have recently attracted attention from scientists investigating EMT's role in drug resistance [90]. Given their centrality to EMT regulation, silencing them may be an efficient way to halt the process. TGF1, NFB, Wnt, Akt, PPAR, and Notch are just a few of the many signaling pathways that play a role in EMT. The renin-angiotensin system (RAS) seems to be involved as well. Some of the methods in which inhibiting these signal transduction might reverse EMT are explored [91]. Recent studies have shown a plethora of microRNAs (miRNAs) that drive or halt EMT in tumors and make cancer cells more sensitive to chemotherapeutics [92, 93]. Post-translational EMT-regulators such as Hakai, FBXW7, and USP27X are emerging as a novel class of therapeutic targets for reversing treatment resistance.

7.5 Conclusion

The EMT's phenotypic variability and plasticity aid in both metastasis and treatment resistance. Molecular insights into the function of EMT in drug resistance have been uncovered via *in vitro* and *in vivo* research in preclinical tumor models and clinical settings in recent years. The investigators have a better grasp on the function of the tumor microenvironment and cellular stemness in the EMT's influence on treatment resistance, as well as on the intermediate E/M states that more properly represent the reality within the tumor. Some scientists believe that treatment strategies based on epithelial plasticity can help patients overcome resistance to therapy. Due to their potential to inhibit both drug resistance and the spread of cancer, plasticity inhibitors are being studied as potential therapeutic interventions in cancer treatment. When combined with chemotherapy and targeted therapy, compounds that target regulators of this plasticity may improve clinical outcomes for cancer patients. Identifying therapeutic targets and new chemosensitizing drugs is necessary to overcome resistance to various chemotherapies. This requires the integration of data from bioinformatics, pharmacogenomics, and chemical genomics. It is hoped that several EMT-related targets will be identified in the not-too-distant future, allowing for the eventual triumph over therapeutic resistance. This creates a new opportunity for the development of therapeutics targeting proteins for which no pharmacological targets have previously been identified.

References

1. Popper, H.H., Progression and metastasis of lung cancer. *Cancer Metastasis Rev.*, 35, 75–91, 2016.
2. Qi, X.K., Han, H.Q., Zhang, H.J. *et al.*, OVOL2 links stemness and metastasis via fine-tuning epithelial-mesenchymal transition in nasopharyngeal carcinoma. *Theranostics*, 8, 2202–16, 2018.
3. Deep, G. and Agarwal, R., Antimetastatic efficacy of silibinin: Molecular mechanisms and therapeutic potential against cancer. *Cancer Metastasis Rev.*, 29, 447–63, 2010.
4. Song, K.A., Niederst, M.J., Lochmann, T.L. *et al.*, Epithelial-to-mesenchymal transition antagonizes response to targeted therapies in lung cancer by suppressing BIM. *Clin. Cancer Res.*, 24, 197–208, 2018.
5. Zeisberg, M. and Neilson, E.G., Biomarkers for epithelial-mesenchymal transitions. *J. Clin. Invest.*, 119, 1429–37, 2009.
6. Thiery, J.P., Acloque, H., Huang, R.Y. *et al.*, Epithelial-mesenchymal transitions in development and disease. *Cell*, 139, 871–90, 2009.
7. Wellner, U., Schubert, J., Burk, U.C. *et al.*, The EMT-activator ZEB1 promotes tumorigenicity by repressing stemness-inhibiting microRNAs. *Nat. Cell Biol.*, 11, 1487–95, 2009.
8. Graham, T.R., Yacoub, R., Taliaferro-Smith, L. *et al.*, Reciprocal regulation of ZEB1 and AR in triple negative breast cancer cells. *Breast Cancer Res. Treat.*, 123, 139–47, 2010.
9. Oliveras-Ferraros, C., Corominas-Faja, B., Cufi, S. *et al.*, Epithelial-to-mesenchymal transition (EMT) confers primary resistance to trastuzumab (Herceptin). *Cell Cycle*, 11, 4020–32, 2012.
10. Ren, J., Chen, Y., Song, H. *et al.*, Inhibition of ZEB1 reverses EMT and chemoresistance in docetaxel-resistant human lung adenocarcinoma cell line. *J. Cell. Biochem.*, 114, 1395–403, 2013.
11. Wilson, C., Nicholes, K., Bustos, D. *et al.*, Overcoming EMT-associated resistance to anti-cancer drugs via Src/FAK pathway inhibition. *Oncotarget*, 5, 7328–41, 2014.
12. Katayama, R., Shaw, A.T., Khan, T.M. *et al.*, Mechanisms of acquired crizotinib resistance in ALK-rearranged lung cancers. *Sci. Transl. Med.*, 4, 120ra17, 2012.
13. Sequist, L.V., Waltman, B.A., Dias-Santagata, D. *et al.*, Genotypic and histological evolution of lung cancers acquiring resistance to EGFR inhibitors. *Sci. Transl. Med.*, 3, 75ra26, 2011.
14. Wilson, C., Ye, X., Pham, T. *et al.*, AXL inhibition sensitizes mesenchymal cancer cells to antimitotic drugs. *Cancer Res.*, 74, 5878–90, 2014.
15. Faber, A.C., Corcoran, R.B., Ebi, H. *et al.*, BIM expression in treatment-naive cancers predicts responsiveness to kinase inhibitors. *Cancer Discovery*, 1, 352–65, 2011.

16. Li, Y., Deutzmann, A., Choi, P.S. *et al.*, BIM mediates oncogene inactivation-induced apoptosis in multiple transgenic mouse models of acute lymphoblastic leukemia. *Oncotarget*, 7, 26926–34, 2016.
17. Karachaliou, N., Codony-Servat, J., Teixido, C. *et al.*, BIM and mTOR expression levels predict outcome to erlotinib in EGFR-mutant non-small-cell lung cancer. *Sci. Rep.*, 5, 17499, 2015.
18. Costa, C., Molina, M.A., Drozdowskyj, A. *et al.*, The impact of EGFR T790M mutations and BIM mRNA expression on outcome in patients with EGFR-mutant NSCLC treated with Erlotinib or chemotherapy in the randomized phase III EURTAC trial. *Clin. Cancer Res.*, 20, 2001–10, 2014.
19. Bean, G.R., Ganesan, Y.T., Dong, Y. *et al.*, PUMA and BIM are required for oncogene inactivation-induced apoptosis. *Sci. Signal.*, 6, ra20, 2013.
20. Ng, K.P., Hillmer, A.M., Chuah, C.T. *et al.*, A common BIM deletion polymorphism mediates intrinsic resistance and inferior responses to tyrosine kinase inhibitors in cancer. *Nat. Med.*, 18, 521–8, 2012.
21. Yochum, Z.A., Cades, J., Wang, H. *et al.*, Targeting the EMT transcription factor TWIST1 overcomes resistance to EGFR inhibitors in EGFR-mutant non-small-cell lung cancer. *Oncogene*, 38, 656–70, 2019.
22. Marcucci, F. and Rumio, C., From "high" ZEB1 to "low" B-cell lymphoma 2-interacting mediator of cell death (BIM)-an epithelial-mesenchymal transition (EMT)-associated drug resistance pathway elucidated. *J. Thorac. Dis.*, 11, 1–5, 2019.
23. Niederst, M.J. and Benes, C.H., EMT twists the road to PI3K. *Cancer Discovery*, 4, 149–51, 2014.
24. Kitai, H., Ebi, H., Tomida, S. *et al.*, Epithelial-to-mesenchymal transition defines feedback activation of receptor tyrosine kinase signaling induced by MEK inhibition in KRAS-mutant lung cancer. *Cancer Discovery*, 6, 754–69, 2016.
25. Zhang, Z., Lee, J.C., Lin, L. *et al.*, Activation of the AXL kinase causes resistance to EGFR-targeted therapy in lung cancer. *Nat. Genet.*, 44, 852–60, 2012.
26. Garinet, S., Didelot, A., Garelli, E. *et al.*, How apoptosis and epithelial-to-mesenchymal transition are nested in EGFR inhibitors resistance in lung cancer. *J. Thorac. Dis.*, 11, 47–9, 2019.
27. Sato, H., Shien, K., Tomida, S. *et al.*, Targeting the miR-200c/LIN28B axis in acquired EGFR-TKI resistance non-small cell lung cancer cells harboring EMT features. *Sci. Rep.*, 7, 40847, 2017.
28. Yue, J., Lv, D., Wang, C. *et al.*, Epigenetic silencing of miR-483-3p promotes acquired gefitinib resistance and EMT in EGFR-mutant NSCLC by targeting integrin beta3. *Oncogene*, 37, 4300–12, 2018.
29. Zheng, X.F., Carstens, J.L., Kim, J., Scheible, M., Kaye, J., Sugimoto, H., Wu, C.C., LeBleu, V.S., Kalluri, R., Epithelial-to-mesenchymal transition is dispensable for metastasis but induces chemoresistance in pancreatic cancer. *Nature*, 527, 525–530, 2015.

30. Teicher, B.A., Holden, S.A., Ara, G., Chen, G., Transforming growth factor-beta in *in vivo* resistance. *Cancer Chemother. Pharmacol.*, 37, 601–609, 1996.
31. Lindner, D., Animal models and the tumor microenvironment: Studies of tumor-host symbiosis. *Semin. Oncol.*, 41, 146–155, 2014.
32. Li, J.P., Liu, H., Yu, J.P., Yu, H.G., Chemoresistance to doxorubicin induces epithelial-mesenchymal transition via upregulation of transforming growth factor signaling in HCT116 colon cancer cells. *Mol. Med. Rep.*, 12, 192–198, 2015.
33. Wu, Y.Y., Ginther, C., Kim, J., Mosher, N., Chung, S.Y., Slamon, D., Vadgama, J.V., Expression of Wnt3 activates Wnt/beta-catenin pathway and promotes EMT-like phenotype in trastuzumab-resistant HER2-overexpressing breast cancer cells. *Mol. Cancer Res.*, 10, 1597–1606, 2012.
34. Della Corte, C.M., Bellevicine, C., Vicidomini, G., Vitagliano, D., Malapelle, U., Accardo, M., Fabozzi, A., Fiorelli, A., Fasano, M., Papaccio, F. *et al.*, SMO gene amplification and activation of the Hedgehog pathway as novel mechanisms of resistance to anti-epidermal growth factor receptor drugs in human lung cancer. *Clin. Cancer Res.*, 21, 4686–4697, 2015.
35. Deng, J.J., Zhang, W., Xu, X.M., Zhang, F., Tao, W.P., Ye, J.J., Ge, W., Twist mediates an aggressive phenotype in human colorectal cancer cells. *Int. J. Oncol.*, 48, 1117–1124, 2016.
36. Zhou, Z.J., Zhang, L., Xie, B.W., Wang, X.P., Yang, X.H., Ding, N.H., Zhang, J., Liu, Q.Q., Tan, G.L., Feng, D.Y. *et al.*, FOXC2 promotes chemoresistance in nasopharyngeal carcinomas via induction of epithelial mesenchymal transition. *Cancer Lett.*, 363, 137–145, 2015.
37. Chiu, W.T., Huang, Y.F., Tsai, H.Y., Chen, C.C., Chang, C.H., Huang, S.C., Hsu, K.F., Chou, C.Y., FOXM1 confers to epithelial-mesenchymal transition, stemness and chemoresistance in epithelial ovarian carcinoma cells. *Oncotarget*, 6, 2349–2365, 2015.
38. Cai, J., Tian, A.X., Wang, Q.S., Kong, P.Z., Du, X., Li, X.Q., Feng, Y.M., FOXF2 suppresses the FOXC2-mediated epithelial mesenchymal transition and multi-drug resistance of basal-like breast cancer. *Cancer Lett.*, 367, 129–137, 2015.
39. Haslehurst, A.M., Koti, M., Dharsee, M., Nuin, P., Evans, K., Geraci, J., Childs, T., Chen, J., Li, J.R., Weberpals, J., Davey, S. *et al.*, EMT transcription factors snail and slug directly contribute to cisplatin resistance in ovarian cancer. *BMC Cancer*, 12, 3–6, 2012.
40. Siebzehnrubl, F.A., Silver, D.J., Tugertimur, B., Deleyrolle, L.P., Siebzehnrubl, D., Sarkisian, M.R., Devers, K.G., Yachnis, A.T., Kupper, M.D., Neal, D. *et al.*, The ZEB1 pathway links glioblastoma initiation, invasion and chemoresistance. *EMBO Mol. Med.*, 5, 1196–1212, 2013.
41. Singh, S.K., Hawkins, C., Clarke, I.D., Squire, J.A., Bayani, J., Hide, T., Henkelman, R.M., Cusimano, M.D., Dirks, P.B., Identification of human brain tumour initiating cells. *Nature*, 432, 396–401, 2004.

42. Huber, M.A., Kraut, N., Beug, H., Molecular requirements for epithelial-mesenchymal transition during tumor progression. *Curr. Opin. Cell Biol.*, 17, 548–558, 2005.
43. Mani, S.A., Guo, W., Liao, M.J., Eaton, E.N., Ayyanan, A., Zhou, A.Y., Brooks, M., Reinhard, F., Zhang, C.C., Shipitsin, M. *et al.*, The epithelial-mesenchymal transition generates cells with properties of stem cells. *Cell*, 133, 704–715, 2008.
44. Singh, A. and Settleman, J., EMT, cancer stem cells and drug resistance: An emerging axis of evil in the war on cancer. *Oncogene*, 29, 4741–4751, 2010.
45. Biddle, A., Liang, X., Gammon, L., Fazil, B., Harper, L.J., Emich, H., Costea, D.E., Mackenzie, I.C., Cancer stem cells in squamous cell carcinoma switch between two distinct phenotypes that are preferentially migratory or proliferative. *Cancer Res.*, 71, 5317–5326, 2011.
46. Liu, S.L., Cong, Y., Wang, D., Sun, Y., Deng, L., Liu, Y.J., Martin-Trevino, R., Shang, L., McDermott, S.P., Landis, M.D. *et al.*, Breast cancer stem cells transition between epithelial and mesenchymal states reflective of their normal counterparts. *Stem Cell Rep.*, 2, 78–91, 2014.
47. Ocana, O.H., Corcoles, R., Fabra, A., Moreno-Bueno, G., Acloque, H., Vega, S., Barrallo-Gimeno, A., Cano, A., Nieto, M.A., Metastatic colonization requires the repression of the epithelial-mesenchymal transition inducer Prrx1. *Cancer Cell*, 22, 709–724, 2012.
48. Gottesman, M.M., Fojo, T., Bates, S.E., Multi-drug resistance in cancer: Role of ATP-dependent transporters. *Nat. Rev. Cancer*, 2, 48–58, 2002.
49. Aller, S.G., Yu, J., Ward, A., Weng, Y., Chittaboina, S., Zhuo, R.P., Harrell, P.M., Trinh, Y.T., Zhang, Q.H., Urbatsch, I.L. *et al.*, Structure of P-plycoprotein reveals a molecular basis for poly-specific drug binding. *Science*, 323, 1718–1722, 2009.
50. Munoz, M., Henderson, M., Haber, M., Norris, M., Role of the MRP1/ABCC1 multi-drug transporter protein in cancer. *IUBMB Life*, 59, 752–757, 2007.
51. Natarajan, K., Xie, Y., Baer, M.R., Ross, D.D., Role of breast cancer resistance protein (BCRP/ABCG2) in cancer drug resistance. *Biochem. Pharmacol.*, 83, 1084–1103, 2012.
52. Saxena, M., Stephens, M.A., Pathak, H., Rangarajan, A., Transcription factors that mediate epithelial-mesenchymal transition lead to multi-drug resistance by upregulating ABC transporters. *Cell Death Dis.*, 2, 2–3, 2011.
53. Uramoto, H., Iwata, T., Onitsuka, T., Shimokawa, H., Hanagiri, T., Oyama, T., Epithelial-mesenchymal transition in EGFR-TKI acquired resistant lung adenocarcinoma. *Anticancer Res.*, 30, 2513–2517, 2010.
54. Lin, Y., Wang, X., Jin, H., EGFR-TKI resistance in NSCLC patients: Mechanisms and strategies. *Am. J. Cancer Res.*, 4, 411–435, 2014.
55. Witta, S.E., Gemmill, R.M., Hirsch, F.R., Coldren, C.D., Hedman, K., Ravdel, L., Helfrich, B., Dziadziuszko, R., Chan, D.C., Sugita, M. *et al.*, Restoring

E-cadherin expression increases sensitivity to epidermal growth factor receptor inhibitors in lung cancer cell lines. *Cancer Res.*, 66, 944–950, 2006.
56. Chang, T.H., Tsai, M.F., Su, K.Y., Wu, S.G., Huang, C.P., Yu, S.L., Yu, Y.L., Lan, C.C., Yang, C.H., Lin, S.B. *et al.*, Slug confers resistance to the epidermal growth factor receptor tyrosine kinase inhibitor. *Am. J. Respir. Crit. Care*, 183, 1071–1079, 2011.
57. Xie, M., He, C.S., Wei, S.H., Zhang, L., Notch-1 contributes to epidermal growth factor receptor tyrosine kinase inhibitor acquired resistance in non-small cell lung cancer *in vitro* and *in vivo*. *Eur. J. Cancer*, 49, 3559–3572, 2013.
58. Soucheray, M., Capelletti, M., Pulido, I., Kuang, Y., Paweletz, C.P., Becker, J.H., Kikuchi, E., Xu, C., Patel, T.B., Al-Shahrour, F. *et al.*, Intratumoral heterogeneity in EGFR-mutant NSCLC results in divergent resistance mechanisms in response to EGFR tyrosine kinase inhibition. *Cancer Res.*, 75, 4372–4383, 2015.
59. Yoshida, T., Song, L., Bai, Y., Kinose, F., Li, J., Ohaegbulam, K.C., Munoz-Antonia, T., Qu, X., Eschrich, S., Uramoto, H. *et al.*, ZEB1 mediates acquired resistance to the epidermal growth factor receptor-tyrosine kinase inhibitors in non-small cell lung cancer. *PLoS One*, 11, e0147344, 2016.
60. Bremnes, R.M., Donnem, T., Al-Saad, S., Al-Shibli, K., Andersen, S., Sirera, R., Camps, C., Marinez, I., Busund, L.T., The role of tumor stroma in cancer progression and prognosis: Emphasis on carcinoma-associated fibroblasts and non-small cell lung cancer. *J. Thorac. Oncol.*, 6, 209–217, 2011.
61. Guan, J., Zhang, H., Wen, Z., Gu, Y.M., Cheng, Y., Sun, Y., Zhang, T.T., Jia, C.W., Lu, Z.H., Chen, J., Retinoic acid inhibits pancreatic cancer cell migration and EMT through the downregulation of IL-6 in cancer associated fibroblast cells. *Cancer Lett.*, 345, 132–139, 2014.
62. Sui, H., Zhu, L., Deng, W., Li, Q., Epithelial-mesenchymal transition and drug resistance: Role, molecular mechanisms, and therapeutic strategies. *Oncol. Res. Treat.*, 37, 584–589, 2014.
63. Jiao, M. and Nan, K.J., Activation of PI3 kinase/Akt/HIF-1 alpha pathway contributes to hypoxia-induced epithelial-mesenchymal transition and chemoresistance in hepatocellular carcinoma. *Int. J. Oncol.*, 40, 461–468, 2012.
64. Bellamy, W.T., P-glycoproteins and multi-drug resistance. *Annu. Rev. Pharmacol.*, 36, 161–183, 1996.
65. Dalton, W.S., Crowley, J.J., Salmon, S.S., Grogan, T.M., Laufman, L.R., Weiss, G.R., Bonnet, J.D., A phase-III randomized study of oral verapamil as a chemosensitizer to reverse drug-resistance in patients with refractory myeloma—A Southwest Oncology Group study. *Cancer*, 75, 815–820, 1995.
66. Kuhnle, M., Egger, M., Muller, C., Mahringer, A., Bernhardt, G., Fricker, G., Konig, B., Buschauer, A., Potent and selective inhibitors of breast cancer resistance protein (ABCG2) derived from the P-glycoprotein (ABCB1) modulator tariquidar. *J. Med. Chem.*, 52, 1190–1197, 2009.

67. Lancet, J.E., Baer, M.R., Duran, G.E., List, A.F., Fielding, R., Marcelletti, J.F., Multani, P.S., Sikic, B.I., A phase I trial of continuous infusion of the multidrug resistance inhibitor zosuquidar with daunorubicin and cytarabine in acute myeloid leukemia. *Leuk. Res.*, 33, 1055–1061, 2009.
68. Gupta, P.B., Onder, T.T., Jiang, G., Tao, K., Kuperwasser, C., Weinberg, R.A., Lander, E.S., Identification of selective inhibitors of cancer stem cells by high-throughput screening. *Cell*, 138, 645–659, 2009.
69. Zhou, Y., Liang, C., Xue, F., Chen, W., Zhi, X., Feng, X., Bai, X., Liang, T., Salinomycin decreases doxorubicin resistance in hepatocellular carcinoma cells by inhibiting the beta-catenin/TCF complex association via FOXO3a activation. *Oncotarget*, 6, 10350–10365, 2015.
70. Hermawan, A., Wagner, E., Roidl, A., Consecutive salinomycin treatment reduces doxorubicin resistance of breast tumor cells by diminishing drug efflux pump expression and activity. *Oncol. Rep.*, 35, 1732–1740, 2016.
71. Toden, S., Okugawa, Y., Jascur, T., Wodarz, D., Komarova, N.L., Buhrmann, C., Shakibaei, M., Boland, C.R., Goel, A., Curcumin mediates chemosensitization to 5-fluorouracil through miRNA-induced suppression of epithelial-to-mesenchymal transition in chemoresistant colorectal cancer. *Carcinogenesis*, 36, 355–367, 2015.
72. Meidhof, S., Brabletz, S., Lehmann, W., Preca, B.T., Mock, K., Ruh, M., Schuler, J., Berthold, M., Weber, A., Burk, U. *et al.*, ZEB1-associated drug resistance in cancer cells is reversed by the class I HDAC inhibitor mocetinostat. *EMBO Mol. Med.*, 7, 831–847, 2015.
73. Namba, T., Kodama, R., Moritomo, S., Hoshino, T., Mizushima, T., Zidovudine, an anti-viral drug, resensitizes gemcitabine-resistant pancreatic cancer cells to gemcitabine by inhibition of the Akt-GSK3 beta-Snail pathway. *Cell Death Discovery*, 6, 1–2, 2015.
74. Evans, J.M., Donnelly, L.A., Emslie-Smith, A.M., Alessi, D.R., Morris, A.D., Metformin and reduced risk of cancer in diabetic patients. *BMJ.*, 330, 1304–1305, 2005.
75. Tomimoto, A., Endo, H., Sugiyama, M., Fujisawa, T., Hosono, K., Takahashi, H., Nakajima, N., Nagashima, Y., Wada, K., Nakagama, H. *et al.*, Metformin suppresses intestinal polyp growth in ApcMin/+ mice. *Cancer Sci.*, 99, 2136–2141, 2008.
76. Jiralerspong, S., Palla, S.L., Giordano, S.H., Meric-Bernstam, F., Liedtke, C., Barnett, C.M., Hsu, L., Hung, M.C., Hortobagyi, G.N., Gonzalez-Angulo, A.M., Metformin and pathologic complete responses to neoadjuvant chemotherapy in diabetic patients with breast cancer. *J. Clin. Oncol.*, 27, 3297–3302, 2009.
77. Hirsch, H.A., Iliopoulos, D., Tsichlis, P.N., Struhl, K., Metformin selectively targets cancer stem cells, and acts together with chemotherapy to block tumor growth and prolong remission. *Cancer Res.*, 69, 7507–7511, 2009.
78. Vazquez-Martin, A., Oliveras-Ferraros, C., Cufi, S., Del Barco, S., Martin-Castillo, B., Menendez, J.A., Metformin regulates breast cancer stem cell

ontogeny by transcriptional regulation of the epithelial-mesenchymal transition (EMT) status. *Cell Cycle*, 9, 3807–3814, 2010.

79. Zhao, Z., Cheng, X., Wang, Y., Han, R., Li, L., Xiang, T., He, L., Long, H., Zhu, B., He, Y., Metformin inhibits the IL-6-induced epithelial-mesenchymal transition and lung adenocarcinoma growth and metastasis. *PLoS One*, 9, e95884, 2014.
80. Qu, C., Zhang, W., Zheng, G., Zhang, Z., Yin, J., He, Z., Metformin reverses multi-drug resistance and epithelial-mesenchymal transition (EMT) via activating AMP-activated protein kinase (AMPK) in human breast cancer cells. *Mol. Cell. Biochem.*, 386, 63–71, 2014.
81. Chou, C.C., Lee, K.H., Lai, I.L., Wang, D., Mo, X., Kulp, S.K., Shapiro, C.L., Chen, C.S., AMPK reverses the mesenchymal phenotype of cancer cells by targeting the Akt-MDM2-Foxo3a signaling axis. *Cancer Res.*, 74, 4783–4795, 2014.
82. Lv, J.F. and Shim, J.S., Existing drugs and their application in drug discovery targeting cancer stem cells. *Arch. Pharm. Res.*, 38, 1617–1626, 2015.
83. Chua, K.N., Sim, W.J., Racine, V., Lee, S.Y., Goh, B.C., Thiery, J.P., A cell-based small molecule screening method for identifying inhibitors of epithelial-mesenchymal transition in carcinoma. *PLoS One*, 7, e33183, 2012.
84. Aref, A.R., Huang, R.Y., Yu, W., Chua, K.N., Sun, W., Tu, T.Y., Bai, J., Sim, W.J., Zervantonakis, I.K., Thiery, J.P. *et al.*, Screening therapeutic EMT blocking agents in a three-dimensional microenvironment. *Integr. Biol.*, 5, 381–389, 2013.
85. Bai, J., Tu, T.Y., Kim, C., Thiery, J.P., Kamm, R.D., Identification of drugs as single agents or in combination to prevent carcinoma dissemination in a microfluidic 3D environment. *Oncotarget*, 6, 36603–36614, 2015.
86. Wen, Z., Feng, S., Wei, L., Wang, Z., Hong, D., Wang, Q., Evodiamine, a novel inhibitor of the Wnt pathway, inhibits the self-renewal of gastric cancer stem cells. *Int. J. Mol. Med.*, 36, 1657–1663, 2015.
87. Xu, L., Zhang, L., Hu, C., Liang, S.J., Fei, X.C., Yan, N.N., Zhang, Y.Y., Zhang, F.C., WNT pathway inhibitor pyrvinium pamoate inhibits the self-renewal and metastasis of breast cancer stem cells. *Int. J. Oncol.*, 48, 1175–1186, 2016.
88. Busaranon, K., Plaimee, P., Sritularak, B., Chanvorachote, P., Moscatilin inhibits epithelial-to-mesenchymal transition and sensitizes anoikis in human lung cancer H460 cells. *J. Nat. Med.*, 70, 18–27, 2016.
89. Zhang, R.R., Zhang, P., Wang, H., Hou, D.M., Li, W.T., Xiao, G.S., Li, C.W., Inhibitory effects of metformin at low concentration on epithelial-mesenchymal transition of CD44(+)CD117(+) ovarian cancer stem cells. *Stem Cell Res. Ther.*, 6, 4–5, 2015.
90. Qin, G., Xu, F., Qin, T., Zheng, Q.F., Shi, D.B., Xia, W., Tian, Y., Tang, Y.L., Wang, J.S., Xiao, X.S. *et al.*, Palbociclib inhibits epithelial-mesenchymal transition and metastasis in breast cancer via c-Jun/COX-2 signaling pathway. *Oncotarget*, 6, 41794–41808, 2015.

91. Xu, B., Jiang, C.W., Han, H.X., Liu, H., Tang, M., Liu, L.X., Ji, W.Y., Lu, X.C., Yang, X.L., Zhang, Y.X. *et al.*, Icaritin inhibits the invasion and epithelial-to-mesenchymal transition of glioblastoma cells by targeting EMMPRIN via PTEN/AKt/HIF-1 alpha signalling. *Clin. Exp. Pharmacol. Physiol.*, 42, 1296–1307, 2015.
92. Han, D., Wu, G., Chang, C., Zhu, F., Xiao, Y., Li, Q.H., Zhang, T., Zhang, L.L., Disulfiram inhibits TGF-beta-induced epithelial-mesenchymal transition and stem-like features in breast cancer via ERK/NF-kappa B/Snail pathway. *Oncotarget*, 6, 40907–40919, 2015.
93. Hseu, Y.C., Huang, Y.C., Korivi, M., Wu, J.J., Way, T.D., Ou, T.T., Chiu, L.W., Lee, C.C., Lin, M.L., Yang, H.L., Zerumbone attenuates TGF-beta 1-mediated epithelial-mesenchymal transition via upregulated E-cadherin expression and downregulated Smad2 signalling pathways in non-small cell lung cancer (A549) cells. *J. Funct. Foods*, 18, 58–72, 2015.

8

Advances in Metallodrug-Driven Combination Therapy for Treatment of Cancer

Rishabha Malviya*, Arun Kumar Singh and Deepika Yadav

Abstract

Cancer is a complex disease that is difficult to understand and cure because it affects many different body systems and activities. Therefore, monotherapy is rarely used to treat cancer. It appears that the use of combination therapy, wherein two or more anticancer drugs are administered at the same time, may be an effective method of treating cancer. It has been shown that the therapeutic efficacy of anticancer drug combinations increases since the drugs work together to target several pathways in a way that is either additive or synergistic. There are a number of compelling benefits to using this strategy, such as lowering the risk of drug resistance, increasing the effectiveness of anticancer treatments by slowing tumor growth, eliminating the ability of cancer cells to spread to new locations, stopping mitotically active cells from dividing, decreasing the number of cancer stem cells, and ensuring that apoptosis is induced in tumors. Most persons with metastatic cancer have a dismal 5-year survival rate. In addition, it takes a lot of time and money to create new cancer treatments. Thus, to acquire the best results at the lowest possible cost, it is best to try out strategies that hit multiple potential survival routes. This chapter details state-of-the-art research into the use of metallodrug-driven combination therapy in the treatment of cancer. Combination therapy including platinum and other metallodrugs is investigated. A conclusion has been reached on the direction of metallodrug-driven combination cancer treatment research and development.

Keywords: Metal complexes, apoptosis, transition metals, cancer, metastasis

**Corresponding author*: rishabhamalviya19@gmail.com

Rishabha Malviya, Arun Kumar Singh and Deepika Yadav. Multi-Drug Resistance in Cancer: Mechanism and Treatment Strategies, (155–170) © 2023 Scrivener Publishing LLC

8.1 Introduction

Human carcinogenesis is a complex process involving many different physiological systems, and the most prevalent hereditary susceptibility to cancer occurs at various points along this process. The spread of a disease, known as metastasis, complicates the treatment of the primary condition. Cancer is notoriously difficult to treat and manage due to the disease's multisystem involvement and metastatic potential [1–4]. The word "cancer" is enough to send shivers down many people's spines because of the lengthy history of human battle with cancer therapy and prevention. Cancer kills more people than any other disease in the world saving cardiovascular disease [5]. Cancer is a leading cause of mortality in the United States, responsible for one in four fatalities each year. The American Cancer Society projects that there will have been 1,762,450 new instances of cancer and 606,880 cancer-related deaths worldwide by the end of 2018. Cancer is the second leading cause of death in Europe, behind only cardiovascular illness (including strokes and heart attacks). The recent cancer fatalities in Europe have been shockingly high (about 20% of deaths). According to Malvezzi *et al.*, there will be 1,410,000 deaths in Europe from cancer this year. Cancer has risen to the position of the second top cause of death in India, possibly due to deteriorating living conditions and a lack of medical resources on the continent [6]. Some of the most often diagnosed cancers in India are those of the lung, breast, colon, rectum, stomach, and liver. Despite this progress, cancer remains a global health crisis. This has resulted in oncologists, medicinal chemists, and biochemists all across the world placing a significant emphasis on cancer therapy. Some of the various procedures used to treat cancer include radiation therapy, chemotherapy, surgery, immunotherapy, and monoclonal antibody therapy. Small molecule medicines (both natural and synthetic) are commonly used in chemotherapy [7]. Chemotherapy plans often take into account cancer's ability to spread to other organs. Chemotherapy, unlike some other treatments, may also reach all of the body's cells and tissues. Chemotherapy is a common method of cancer treatment that employs a broad variety of anticancer medicines and medication combinations.

Humans have known that certain metals have therapeutic properties for at least the last five thousand years. Several substances containing metal ions/atoms are used therapeutically for the treatment of different illnesses, including bacterial and fungal infections, viral infections, and cancer, or so the claim goes. Metal compounds (metal complexes) are physiologically active because of their interesting binding characteristics with essential biomolecules including proteins and hormones [8]. Furthermore, enzymes and nucleic acids contribute to the growth and metastasis of cancer cells.

As far as inorganic medicinal chemistry goes, metal complexes are now the gold standard. The use of metal complexes in drug design provides a significant lot of versatility (metallodrugs). Modifying the core metal ion or atom and its oxidation state can optimize the kinetic and thermodynamic features of metal complexes [9, 10]. When it comes to the bioactivity of metal complexes, both the metal center and the ligand structure are crucial factors. The most widely recognized metallodrug for cancer treatment is cisplatin (Figure 8.1). Peyrone has initially synthesized cisplatin in 1844. In 1965, while investigating the effects of ac on *E. coli* development, Rosenberg and his colleagues made the surprising discovery that ac had anticancer properties. Cisplatin was approved for use in the treatment of testicular and ovarian malignancies thanks to the efforts of Prof. Rosenberg's research group. So far, cisplatin has proven to be the most effective treatment for testicular, ovarian, bladder, cervical, head and neck, small cell, and non-small cell lung cancers.

Research and development of novel metallodrugs were sparked by the announcement of the accidental discovery of cisplatin. Contrarily, research

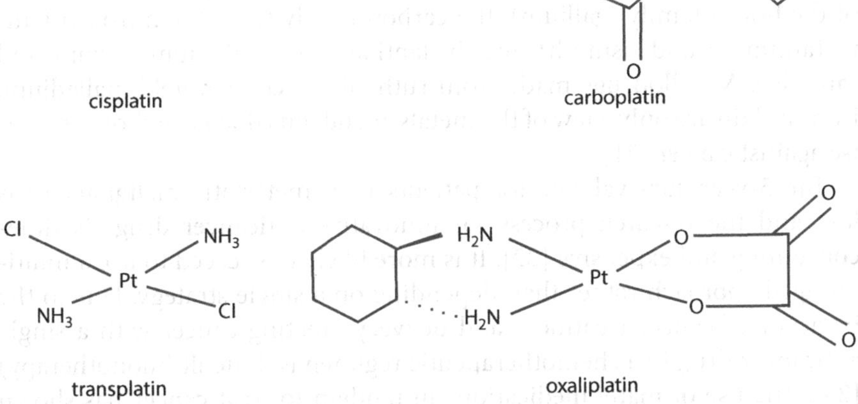

Figure 8.1 Chemical structure of cisplatin complex.

shows that cisplatin has several unfavorable side effects, including ototoxicity (balance/hearing loss), neurotoxicity, renal impairment, and more. Medical inorganic chemists should have sought cisplatin substitutes among other metallodrugs. New cisplatin analogues have been created that are more effective against cancer than cisplatin while having fewer side effects. The children of cisplatin were then created; they include carboplatin, oxaliplatin, and necaplatin [11, 12].

The cancers of the ovary, the lung, and the head and neck have all responded effectively to carboplatin therapy. Treatment of adjuvant and metastatic colorectal cancer with oxaliplatin, 5-fluorouracil (5-FU), and folinic acid has been demonstrated to be effective [13–15]. Head and neck, esophageal, non-small cell lung, and small cell lung cancers were all treated with nedaplatin. "The third-generation cisplatin analogues heptaplatin and lobaplatin are shown in Figure 8.1. The use of heptaplatin has shown promising results in the treatment of both gastric cancer and chronic myelogenous leukemia [16–18]. Metastatic breast and lung cancers respond well to lobaplatin, a platinum-based chemotherapy medication. The increasing prevalence of medication resistance as a result of cisplatin treatment failures has led to a rise in the popularity of alternative medicines. This has led to the creation of a variety of platinum complexes featuring altered structures and shown promise against cancer. Potential platinum metallodrug treatments have increased in number. Nonplatinum anticancer metallodrugs were developed due to the limitations of platinum-based anticancer metallodrugs [19, 20]. As a result, a wide variety of anticancer metallodrugs utilizing a wide range of metal ions/atoms besides platinum have been produced. This class of ions includes the first and second transition metals, as well as the lanthanides (lanthanum and neodymium), members of the boron family (gallium), the carbon family (tin), the nitrogen family (antimony and bismuth), and the lanthanides (lanthanum, cerium, and samariu). Metallodrugs made from ruthenium, copper, gold, palladium, iron, and tin are only a few of the metals/metal ions that have shown promise against cancer [21].

The 5-year survival rate for patients with metastatic malignancies is low, and the research process for innovative anticancer drugs is time-consuming and expensive [22]. It is more likely to succeed to use a multi-pronged approach rather than depending on a single strategy. Due to the intricacy of cancer treatment and delivery, treating cancer with a single anticancer drug in a chemotherapeutic regimen is difficult (monotherapy) [23]. The use of many medications in tandem to treat cancer has shown some promise.

The synergistic or cumulative effects of numerous medicines are responsible for the enhanced therapeutic results that occur when many medications are administered together. Increases anticancer efficacy and decreases resistance by suppressing tumor development, preventing metastasis, and eliminating cancer cells by apoptosis (inducing the death of cancer cells) [24]. There has been increasing research interest in the use of metallodrugs in combination treatment for cancer over the past two decades, as shown by a review of the available data. The urgent need for new and improved anticancer therapies may be contributing to this heightened interest. There is a dearth of literature on the use of metallodrugs in conjunction with chemotherapy [25–28]. The purpose of this chapter is to present an up-to-date overview of metallodrugs' applications in cancer therapy and to discuss how they may be used with other treatment approaches for enhanced efficacy. This chapter will discuss the potential of metallodrugs in conjunction with other anticancer drugs. The use of platinum and other metallodrugs in a combination treatment setting is evaluated. The future of research and development of metallodrug-driven combination cancer treatments has been decided [29].

8.2 Cancer Treatment Using Combination Therapy

The practice of utilizing many therapies all at once is often referred to as "polytherapy." Employing more than one therapeutic method (or "modality") in the treatment of a patient's condition. The use of two or more anticancer medications to specifically target cancer-inducing or cell-sustaining pathways is the basis of combination therapy, which is widely used in cancer treatment. A combination of chemotherapeutic medications was not proposed for the treatment of acute leukemia until 1965, headed by a team of researchers including Emil Frei, James F. Holland, and Emil J. Freireich. The POMP regimen was used to treat pediatric acute lymphocytic leukemia (methotrexate, 6-mercaptopurine, vincristine, and prednisone). Both tumor burden and duration of remission were reduced by the combination treatment regimen. The encouraging outcomes of combination therapy based on POMP have given the required push for further research into synergistic or additive effects. Multiple studies have demonstrated that combined chemotherapy may have synergistic or cumulative effects. Antibiotic minocycline, which has demonstrated anticancer benefits in the past, and the pan-Bcl-2 inhibitor sabutoclax have been discovered to have a synergistic effect on the intrinsic apoptotic pathway [30]. Moreover, pancreatic ductal adenocarcinoma was found to be selectively toxic and to prevent tumor development in both *in vitro* and *in vivo* investigations [31, 32]. Thus, the administration of many anticancer medications at once, each of which targets a distinct biological route, may have additive or synergistic effects. Numerous forms of cancer are still often treated with monotherapy. But it is generally considered less effective than combination therapy. Monotherapy is not selective and so mostly kills rapidly dividing cells. Both healthy and cancerous cells will be destroyed as a result of this. It is common knowledge that chemotherapy presents the patient with a multitude of risks and adverse effects. Chemotherapy has been shown to have deleterious effects on bone marrow cells, making patients more susceptible to host infections [33]. By targeting multiple biological pathways at once, combination therapy has the potential to reduce toxicity even when one of the drugs utilized is cytotoxic [34]. Therefore, the drug combination results in a decreased dosage of each individual treatment.

Current thinking suggests that combination treatment may reduce the toxicity of chemotherapy medicines on healthy cells while maintaining their cytotoxic effects on cancer cells. Normal cells are usually protected from becoming cytotoxic by drug combination regimens that are antagonistic to one another (in terms of their impact on normal cells). According to Professor Blagosklonny, the therapeutic effectiveness of cancer therapy increases when combined with other treatments. Z-DEVD-fmk, an apoptosis-inducing drug, was used in conjunction with it. Z-DEVD-fmk was proven to be ineffective against cancer cells expressing p-glycoprotein, however, the apoptosis-inducing chemical still caused apoptosis to occur in these cells. Z-DEVD-fmk, on the other hand, had an immediate effect on the vast majority of non-p-glycoprotein-containing normal cells, causing them to revert back to apoptosis [35].

There has been a recent explosion in the study of drug combinations for the treatment of cancer, with both novel and established anticancer medicines being evaluated in a wide range of potential drug combination regimens.

8.3 Combined Treatment with Metallodrugs for Cancer Treatment

The potential of palladium and other metallodrugs as cancer treatments has been intensively researched. Nonplatinum anticancer drugs based on ruthenium or a copper metal core have also had substantial success on the market despite being less expensive than platinum-based therapies.

8.3.1 Platinum Metallodrugs

However, the great majority of anticancer medicines are organic molecules, and just a tiny proportion are metallodrugs like platinum metallodrugs like cisplatin. When it comes to metallodrugs used to treat cancer, cisplatin has been around the longest and is the most well-known for the longest time. Despite the fact that cisplatin research began in 1844, it was not until 1978 that it was widely used in the clinic to treat cancer [36]. Platinum metallodrugs like cisplatin, carboplatin, and oxaliplatin are only a few of the alternatives available for treating cancer. Changing Cl concentrations inside the cell activate most platinum drugs, which bind DNA and halt normal cell cycle progression and transcription. Due to their high cytotoxicity toward human host cells, platinum metallodrugs show promise as a potential cancer treatment. The problem of acquired or intrinsic drug resistance to platinum therapy may be overcome by the use of many treatments, each of which targets a distinct pharmacological route. Clinical studies have demonstrated the superiority of combination therapy over single-drug treatments for many different kinds of cancer [37].

The FDA has also approved fluorouracil and folinic acid for the treatment of advanced testicular, ovarian, and bladder cancers. When used with other FDA-approved therapies, the second-generation platinum drug carboplatin has been demonstrated to be helpful in the treatment of ovarian cancer [38]. When used in conjunction with other chemotherapy drugs, oxaliplatin, a metallodrug developed in the second half of the 20th century, can be highly successful in the treatment of colon and lung cancer. In Japan, where it has been approved for use, nedaplatin has been widely used in combination therapies as an alternate treatment for urological cancers. First-line treatments for small-cell lung cancer in the United States have consistently included VP-16 and cisplatin since the 1980s. Etoposide, paclitaxel, and topotecan were used together in a phase study for the treatment of small-cell lung cancer [39]. While the potential benefits of combining these three therapies are acknowledged, the possibility of undesirable side effects cannot be discounted. Patients with advanced gastric cancer often get cisplatin and 5-fluorouracil (5-FU) chemotherapy doublets (AGC).

Currently, it is uncertain which treatment approach is best for AGC. Innovative chemotherapeutic drugs such as oral 5FU, taxanes, and irinotecan have been demonstrated to enhance outcomes when administered either as a single agent or in combination with nonplatinum-based chemotherapy, however, it is not yet known if these treatments should be used to treat patients with AGC. Metallodrugs and nanomaterials have been connected by several studies to more effective cancer medicine formulations.

Current anticancer drugs may be replaced in the future by metal-based treatments and combinations, according to the same study's theory [40].

The anticancer effectiveness of platinum treatments is improved by encapsulation in different nanoparticles, and the problem of their sluggish diffusion is resolved. Nanocarrier delivery is a viable approach because of the toxicity and lack of target specificity of platinum medicines. Researchers have studied a wide variety of nanocarriers. Increased loading of platinum treatments and improved distribution to specific sites employing nanocarriers built of gold or lipoic acid have been examined for their potential to minimize cytotoxicity [41]. Recent research into the molecular mechanism of action of platinum anticancer drugs has shown a novel approach to increasing their effectiveness and selectivity in a protein nanocage.

For at least the past five thousand years, people have recognized that some metals may be used for medical purposes. The medicinal use of various compounds containing metal ions/atoms has been proposed for the treatment of many diseases, including but not limited to bacterial and fungal infections, viral infections, and cancer [42]. Some metal compounds (metal complexes) have remarkable binding capabilities with crucial biomolecules like proteins and hormones, making them physiologically active. In addition, enzymes and nucleic acids promote cancer cell growth and metastasis.

There has been a paradigm shift in inorganic medicinal chemistry, with metal complexes taking center stage. Metal complexes provide a great deal of flexibility in medication creation (metallodrugs). The kinetic and thermodynamic properties of metal complexes can be optimized by altering the core metal ion or atom and its oxidation state [43]. Both the metal center and the ligand structure play important roles in the bioactivity of metal complexes. Cisplatin is the best-known metallodrug used to treat cancer. Prof. Rosenberg's research team successfully advocated for cisplatin's use in treating testicular and ovarian cancers. Testicular, ovarian, bladder, cervical, head and neck, small cell, and non-small cell lung cancers have all shown remarkable responses to cisplatin.

The news of the accidental discovery of cisplatin prompted interest in the study and creation of new metallodrugs. Contrarily, studies suggest that cisplatin has a number of unfavorable side effects, such as ototoxicity (balance/hearing loss), neurotoxicity, renal impairment, and more. They should have looked for alternatives to cisplatin among other metallodrugs, say medical inorganic chemists. There are now cisplatin analogues that are more potent than cisplatin against cancer yet has fewer adverse effects. The offspring of cisplatin are the analogues carboplatin, oxaliplatin, and necaplatin.

Carboplatin treatment has shown promising results in treating ovarian, lung, and head and neck malignancies. There is evidence that oxaliplatin, 5-fluorouracil (5-FU), and folinic acid are useful in treating adjuvant and metastatic colorectal cancer [44]. Nedaplatin has been used for the treatment of malignancies of the head and neck, esophagus, non-small cell lung, and small cell lung. Figure 8.1 displays heptaplatin and lobaplatin, third-generation cisplatin analogs. Both gastric cancer and chronic myelogenous leukemia have responded well to heptaplatin therapy. Lobaplatin, a platinum-based chemotherapeutic drug, is effective against metastatic breast and lung malignancies. There has been a growth in the use of alternative medications due to the rising prevalence of drug resistance as a result of the failure of cisplatin therapy [45]. This has resulted in the development of several platinum complexes with modified structures that have exhibited anticancer activity. More and more platinum metallodrug therapies have shown promise. In response to the shortcomings of platinum-based anticancer metallodrugs, newer, nonplatinum-based metallodrugs have been created. This has led to the development of several metallodrugs with anticancer activity that utilize a wide range of metal ions/atoms in addition to platinum. Members of the boron family (gallium), the carbon family (tin), the nitrogen family (antimony and bismuth), and the lanthanides (lanthanum and neodymium) are all included in this group of ions (lanthanum, cerium, and samariu). Several metals and metal ions, including those found in metallodrugs, have demonstrated activity against cancer.

Patients with metastatic cancers have a poor 5-year survival rate, and developing new anticancer treatments is a costly and time-consuming endeavor. Rather than relying on a single technique, it is preferable to employ a multifaceted approach. It is challenging to treat cancer with a single anticancer agent in a chemotherapeutic regimen because of the complexity of cancer treatment and delivery (monotherapy). There has been some success in treating cancer using a combination of drugs.

Improved therapeutic results arise when many medications are provided at once due to the synergistic or cumulative effects of these drugs [46]. Boosts the effectiveness of anticancer treatments and reduces patient resistance by inhibiting tumor growth, blocking metastasis, and killing cancer cells via apoptosis (inducing the death of cancer cells). A look at the available data reveals that the use of metallodrugs in combination with cancer treatment has garnered increased attention from researchers over the past two decades. This increased focus may be influenced by the pressing demand for cutting-edge cancer treatments. Combining chemotherapy with metallodrugs is an area where there is a paucity of published research. This chapter's goal is to provide readers with an up-to-date summary of metallodrugs' uses in cancer therapy and to explore how these drugs might be used with others to improve treatment outcomes. The potential of metallodrugs in combination with other anticancer drugs will be discussed in this chapter. Platinum and other metallodrugs are assessed for their potential application in a multimodal therapeutic context. The development of metallodrug-driven combination cancer therapies will continue in the future.

However, despite clinical research assessing the effectiveness of FDA-approved pharmaceutical combinations in populations with varying genetic make-up, significant inter-patient variation persists. Results from clinical trials with drug combinations have been all over the map. Even if the other drug(s) in the combination are less effective in treating the patient's cancer, some patients benefit more from that therapy than others [47].

As a result, the ultimate goal of cancer research is to determine which pharmacological combinations may improve patient outcomes by acting on certain malignancies in an additive or synergistic manner. Future research in this field may be directed by biomarker-guided clinical trials, computational modelling, clinical data, and studies based on these biomarkers. Alternating between medications as the disease advances may also improve the efficacy of the combination drugs a patient takes.

8.4 Nonplatinum Metallodrugs

Despite the fact that platinum drugs are used in over half of all chemotherapy plans, platinum resistance is becoming a major clinical issue. This has led to the development of new, non-platinum chemotherapy drugs, which differ from platinum-based therapies by having a more targeted and selective effect on cancer cells [48]. The chemical similarities amongst platinum metals have contributed to a rise in interest in ruthenium (II/III) complexes (Pt, Pd, Rh, Ir, Ru, and Os). Several metal complexes have been developed to address the issue of platinum resistance; nevertheless, ruthenium-based compounds are widely held to be the most effective. Numerous attempts have been made to produce ruthenium complexes; however, just a handful (RM175, RAPTA-C, NAMI-A, KP1019/NKP1339, and TLD1433) have progressed through clinical trials and are now being researched as chemotherapeutic medications. The octahedral Ru(II) complex TLD1433 has the potential for application in photodynamic treatment.

In their research, Berger and colleagues looked at the relationship between ruthenium compounds and standard cancer treatments.

The combination of KP1339 with sorafenib for the treatment of hepatocellular carcinoma (Hep3B) had better outcomes than either medicine used alone. The median survival time for patients was enhanced by 3.9-fold when KP1339 and sorafenib were used together, compared to 2.4- and 1.9-fold when used separately [49]. Sorafenib-resistant tumor cells were also effectively suppressed by this combination. After investigating further, scientists realized that the combination not only boosted their intracellular concentration but also messed with DNA synthesis, rendering mitosis impossible and increasing apoptosis induction. Combining NAMI-A with gemcitabine effectively suppressed non-small cell lung cancer cells in clinical studies, but it also caused serious adverse effects, such as neutropenia, anemia, and renal impairment.

It has been suggested that new medication combinations can be discovered through high-throughput screening. The anticancer effects of doxorubicin and NAMI-A are amplified when used together [50]. The breast cancer drug doxorubicin accumulated more rapidly in those using NAMI-A. Evidence from *in vivo* studies using mouse MCA mammary cancer showed that this combination considerably enhanced the ability to suppress tumor spread. In a preclinical model of lung metastasis, this combination demonstrated promise synergistic benefits despite substantial adverse effects at maximum dosages. Combination therapy with doxorubicin and the RAPTA-C ruthenium complex increased the rate of apoptosis in A2780 ovarian cancer cells compared to either medication alone. Apoptosis-driven normalization of tumor vasculature reduces vascular extravasations, allowing oxygen-dependent phototherapy to work more effectively [51].

These investigations have established a causal relationship between anti-angiogenesis and anticancer properties. RuCl2(KTZ)2 is a chemical that was created by combining ketoconazole (KTZ), a second-line anticancer drug, with ruthenium, which is used to treat hormone-resistant cancers. The combination of these two medicines greatly increased caspase-3 expression and induced cell death in the C8161 melanoma cell line. The use of ruthenium complexes in conjunction with photoacoustic (PA) imaging has greatly facilitated tumor identification and therapy. Combinations of ruthenium compounds with other anticancer medicines have shown promising outcomes. Human endothelial (ECRF24 and HUVEC) and ovarian cancer (A2780 and A2780cisR) cell viability was significantly reduced when RAPTA-C was combined with the EGFR inhibitor erlotinib. Erlotinib increased RAPTA-C absorption into human ovarian cancer cells compared to RAPTA-C monotherapy, but not into endothelial cells. The presence of chromosomal bridges that survive mitotic exit and prolong abscission is associated with cellular senescence in A2780 and A2780cisR. However, no combination of copper and gold metal complexes has been examined or authorized by the FDA, despite the fact that both compounds individually show promise as anticancer treatments [51].

8.5 Conclusion

Several medicines that aim to interrupt particular cancer-causing pathways have been developed in recent decades. Combination treatments have led to some of the most promising breakthroughs in the war against cancer. Because cancer cells are often unable to adapt to the cytotoxic effects of various drugs being delivered at once, combination treatment offers the potential to target multiple pathways and prevent drug resistance. The disruption of homeostasis is a contributing element in the rapid multiplication of cancer cells. The cell cycle is generally arrested in response to DNA damage by tumor suppressor genes like p53, which are frequently mutated in malignancies. These alterations can promote the growth of cancerous cells. Tumor suppressor gene alterations cause more DNA damage and less cell cycle arrest, which fuels the growth of cancer cells and makes the tumor more aggressive. Autocrine growth factors and the activation of the autocrine loop contribute to the proliferation of cancer cells. To control cancer and the danger of cancer cells becoming more aggressive and incurable, several drug combinations targeting distinct pathways may be used. Monotherapy treatment methods cannot reduce the severity of side effects since the amount of the drugs cannot be lowered. Targeting the tumor's heterogeneity with combination therapy improves the odds that all cancer cell types, including the cancer stem cells that cause drug resistance and cancer recurrence after remission in later years, will be eliminated.

Many studies have demonstrated positive outcomes from using combination therapies, but there are also serious drawbacks to consider. When many drugs are used together, however, they can increase the risk of serious adverse effects. Because of this, it can be challenging to isolate the offending drug or drugs, and even more so to establish which drug(s) should have their dosage reduced. When drugs with similar mechanisms of action and toxicities are used together, the resulting clinical symptoms and toxicities could be more severe, thereby affecting patients' life expectancy. Combination therapy can have negative effects on a patient's finances and mental health if the side effects are not managed effectively. It is crucial to take into account possible drug interactions while designing a combination therapy regimen for the treatment of cancer. The optimal medicine combination would have maximum efficacy with minimal side effects.

The several metallodrugs now under development and on the market are discussed in this chapter as prospective therapeutic options. Oncologists from all over the world are interested in cancer therapy metallodrugs because they have demonstrated economic benefits in clinical settings. Metal-based medication combinations have been found to be more efficient and effective than those used alone. In most cases, the efficacy and efficacy of decreasing drug resistance of metallodrugs are both increased by their use as part of a combined or synergistic therapy.

References

1. Norn, S., Permin, H., Kruse, E., Kruse, P.R., Mercury a major agent in the history of medicine and alchemy. *Dan Medicinhist Årboq.*, 36, 21–40, 2008.
2. Agnew, J., *Medicine in the Old West: A history, 1850–1900*, McFarland, Jefferson, NC, 2010.
3. Waxman, S. and Anderson, K.C., History of the development of arsenic derivatives in cancer therapy. *Oncologist*, 6, Suppl 2, 3–10, 2001.
4. Fricker, S.P., Medical uses of gold compounds. *Gold Bull.*, 29, 2, 53–60, 1996.
5. Jungwirth, U., Kowol, C.R., Keppler, B.K., Hartinger, C.G., Berger, W., Heffeter, P., Anticancer activity of metal complexes: Involvement of redox processes. *Antioxid. Redox Signal.*, 15, 4, 1085–1127, 2011.
6. Nicolini, M., *Platinum and other metal coordination compounds in cancer chemotherapy*, vol. 54, Springer, New York, 1997.
7. Ji, H.-F., Li, X.-J., Zhang, H.-Y., Natural products and drug discovery. Can thousands of years of ancient medical knowledge lead us to new and powerful drug combinations in the fight against cancer and dementia? *EMBO Rep.*, 10, 3, 194–200, 2009.
8. Frezza, M., Hindo, S., Chen, D. *et al.*, Novel metals and metal complexes as platforms for cancer therapy. *Curr. Pharm. Des.*, 16, 16, 1813–1825, 2010.
9. Bruijnincx, P. and Sadler, P., New trends for metal complexes with anticancer activity. *Curr. Opin. Chem. Biol.*, 12, 12, 197–206, 2008.
10. Mourino, V., Cattalini, J.P., Boccaccini, A.R., Metallic ions as therapeutic agents in tissue engineering scaffolds: An overview of their biological applications and strategies for new developments. *J. R. Soc. Interface*, 9, 68, 401–419, 2012.
11. Benedetti, B.T., Peterson, E.J., Kabolizadeh, P., Martínez, A., Kipping, R., Farrell, N.P., Effects of noncovalent platinum drug–protein interactions on drug efficacy: Use of fluorescent conjugates as probes for drug metabolism. *Mol. Pharm.*, 8, 3, 940–948, 2011.

12. Bhargava, A. and Vaishampayan, U.N., Satraplatin: Leading the new generation of oral platinum agents. *Expert Opin. Investig. Drugs*, 18, 11, 1787–1797, 2009.
13. Milacic, V., Fregona, D., Dou, Q.P., Gold complexes as prospective metal-based anticancer drugs. *Histol. Histopathol.*, 23, 1, 101–108, 2008.
14. Bindoli, A., Pia, M., Scutari, G., Gabbiani, C., Casini, A., Messori, L., Thioredoxin reductase: A target for gold compounds acting as potential anticancer drugs. *Coord. Chem. Rev.*, 253, 1692–1707, 2009.
15. Kostova, I., Ruthenium complexes as anticancer agents. *Curr. Med. Chem.*, 13, 9, 1085–1107, 2006.
16. Karlenius, T.C. and Tonissen, K.F., Thioredoxin and cancer: A role for thioredoxin in all states of tumor oxygenation. *Cancers (Basel)*, 2, 2, 209–232, 2010.
17. Arredondo, M. and Núñez, M.T., Iron and copper metabolism. *Mol. Aspects Med.*, 26, 4–5, 313–327, 2005.
18. Balamurugan, K. and Schaffner, W., Copper homeostasis in eukaryotes: Teetering on a tightrope. *Biochim. Biophys. Acta*, 1763, 7, 737–746, 2006.
19. Go, Y.M. and Jones, D.P., Redox compartmentalization in eukaryotic cells. *Biochim. Biophys. Acta*, 1780, 11, 1273–1290, 2008.
20. Gupte, A. and Mumper, R.J., Elevated copper and oxidative stress in cancer cells as a target for cancer treatment. *Cancer Treat. Rev.*, 35, 1, 32–46, 2009.
21. Hentze, M.W., Muckenthaler, M.U., Andrews, N.C., Balancing acts: Molecular control of mamalian iron metabolism. *Cell*, 117, 3, 285–297, 2004.
22. Pattan, S.R., Pawar, S.B., VEtal, S.S., Gharate, U.D., Bhawar, S.B., The scope of metal complexes in drug design – A review. *Indian Drugs*, 49, 11, 5–12, 2012.
23. Haas, K.L. and Franz, K.J., Application of metal coordination chemistry to explore and manipulate cell biology. *Chem. Rev.*, 109, 10, 4921–4960, 2010.
24. Yan, Y.K., Melchart, M., Habtemariam, A., Sadler, P.J., Organometallic chemistry, biology and medicine: Ruthenium arene anticancer complexes. *Chem. Commun.*, 14, 38, 4764–4776, 2005.
25. Salga, M.S., Ali, H.M., Abdulla, M.A., Abdelwahab, S.I., Acute oral toxicity evaluations of some zinc(II) complexes derived from 1-(2-Salicylaldiminoethyl) piperazine schiff bases in rats. *Int. J. Mol. Sci.*, 13, 2, 1393–1404, 2012.
26. Florea, A.-M. and Büsselberg, D., Cisplatin as an anti-tumor drug: Cellular mechanisms of activity, drug resistance and induced side effects. *Cancers (Basel)*, 3, 1, 1351–1371, 2011.
27. Monneret, C., Platinum anticancer drugs. From serendipity to rational design. *Ann. Pharm. Fr.*, 69, 6, 286–295, 2011.
28. Chan, B.A. and Coward, J.I.G., Review article chemotherapy advances in small-cell lung cancer. *J. Thorac. Dis.*, 5, 5, S565–S578, 2007.
29. Uehara, T., Yamate, J., Torii, M., Maruyama, T., Comparative nephrotoxicity of cisplatin and nedaplatin: Mechanisms and histopathological characteristics. *J. Toxicol. Pathol.*, 24, 2, 87–94, 2011.

30. Johnstone, T.C., Suntharalingam, K., Lippard, S.J., The next generation of platinum drugs: Targeted Pt(II) agents, nanoparticle delivery, and Pt(IV) prodrugs. *Chem. Rev.*, 116, 5, 3436–3486, 2016.
31. Peng, Y., Liu, Y.E., Ren, X.C. *et al.*, A phase I clinical trial of dose escalation of lobaplatin in combination with fixed - Dose docetaxel for the treatment of human solid tumours that had progressed following chemotherapy. *Oncol. Lett.*, 9, 1, 67–74, 2015.
32. Shah, N. and Dizon, D.S., New-generation platinum agents for solid tumors. *Future Oncol.*, 5, 1, 33–42, 2009.
33. Karlin, D.A., Breitz, H.B., Weiden, P.I., Use of picoplatin to treat colorectal cancer. *United States Patent Application Publication*, 1, 1–19, 2012.
34. Wheate, N.J., Walker, S., Craig, G.E., Oun, R., The status of platinum anticancer drugs in the clinic and in clinical trials. *Dalton Trans.*, 39, 35, 8113–8127, 2010.
35. Liu, D., Poon, C., Lu, K., He, C., Lin, W., Self-assembled nanoscale coordination polymers with trigger release properties for effective anticancer therapy. *Nat. Commun.*, 25, 5, 4182, 2014.
36. Apps, M.G., Choi, E.H., Wheate, N.J., The state-of-play and future of platinum drugs. *Endocr. Relat. Cancer*, 22, 4, R219–R233, 2015.
37. Ohi, H., Ashizaki, M., Obata, M. *et al.*, Syntheses, characterization, and antitumor activities of platinum(II) and palladium(II) complexes with sugar-conjugated triazole ligands. *Chem. Biodivers.*, 9, 9, 1903–1915, 2012.
38. Mi, Q., Ma, Y., Gao, X. *et al.*, 2-Deoxyglucose conjugated platinum(II) complexes for targeted therapy: Design, synthesis, and antitumor activity. *J. Biomol. Struct. Dyn.*, 34, 1–12, 2015.
39. Patra, M., Johnstone, T.C., Suntharalingam, K., Lippard, S.J., A potent glucose-platinum conjugate exploits glucose transporters and preferentially accumulates in cancer cells. *Angew. Chem. Int. Ed. Engl.*, 55, 7, 2550–2554, 2016.
40. Ellena, J., Gozzo, C., Cominetti, M.R. *et al.*, Chiral platinum(II) complexes featuring phosphine and chloroquine ligands as cytotoxic and monofunctional DNA-binding agents. *Inorg. Chem.*, 54, 24, 11709–11720, 2015.
41. Timothy, C., Wilson, J.J., Lippard, S.J., Link, C., Monofunctional and higher-valent platinum anticancer agents. *Inorg. Chem.*, 52, 21, 12234–12249, 2013.
42. Coluccia, M. and Natile, G., Trans-platinum complexes in cancer therapy. *Anticancer Agents Med. Chem.*, 7, 111–23, 2007.
43. Abu-Surrah, A.S. and Kettunen, M., Platinum group antitumor chemistry: Design and development of new anticancer drugs complementary to cisplatin. *Curr. Med. Chem.*, 13, 1337–57, 2006.
44. Lin, X., Okuda, T., Holzer, A., Howell, S.B., The copper transporter CTR1 regulates cisplatin uptake in Saccharomyces cerevisiae. *Mol. Pharmacol.*, 62, 1154–9, 2002.

45. Fuertes, M.A., Alonso, C., Perez, J.M., Biochemical modulation of Cisplatin mechanisms of action: Enhancement of antitumor activity and circumvention of drug resistance. *Chem. Rev.*, 103, 645–62, 2003.
46. Jennerwein, M. and Andrews, P.A., Effect of intracellular chloride on the cellular pharmacodynamics of cis-diamminedichloroplatinum(II). *Drug Metab. Dispos.*, 23, 178–84, 1995.
47. Legendre, F., Bas, V., Kozelka, J., Chottard, J.C., A complete kinetic study of GG versus AG plantination suggests that the doubly aquated derivatives of cisplatin are the actual DNA binding species. *Chemistry.*, 6, 2002–10, 2000.
48. Pizarro, A.M. and Sadler, P.J., Unusual DNA binding modes for metal anticancer complexes. *Biochimie*, 91, 1198–211, 2009.
49. Knox, R.J., Friedlos, F., Lydall, D.A., Roberts, J.J., Mechanism of cytotoxicity of anticancer platinum drugs: Evidence that cisdiamminedichloroplatinum(II) and cis-diammine-(1,1-cyclobutanedicarboxylato)platinum(II) differ only in the kinetics of their interaction with DNA. *Cancer Res.*, 46, 1972–9, 1986.
50. Jakupec, M.A., Galanski, M., Keppler, B.K., Tumour-inhibiting platinum complexes–state of the art and future perspectives. *Rev. Physiol. Biochem. Pharmacol.*, 146, 1–54, 2003.
51. Wang, D. and Lippard, S.J., Cellular processing of platinum anticancer drugs. *Nat. Rev. Drug Discovery*, 4, 307–20, 2005.

9

Novel Strategies Preventing Emergence of MDR in Breast Cancer

Rishabha Malviya*, Arun Kumar Singh and Deepika Yadav

Abstract

When it comes to female cancers, breast cancer is both the most prevalent and the deadliest. Unfortunately, the efficacy of current chemotherapies in treating later stages of breast cancer is decreasing. To a considerable extent, drug efflux transporters like P-glycoprotein cause the MDR phenotype, an important chemoresistance mechanism. Natural selection and chemotherapeutic treatment are two potential drivers of multi-drug resistance (MDR). This mechanism of chemoresistance must be thoroughly investigated and addressed since chemotherapy is the backbone of treatment for advanced-stage triple-negative breast cancer and is often included in regimens for other advanced-stage subtypes of breast cancer. Efflux transporters for drugs will be the focus of this chapter as the author learn how they contribute to chemoresistance in breast cancer. To achieve this end, researchers will look at nanotherapeutic techniques and prospective drugs that might mitigate the consequences of multi-drug resistance.

Keywords: Drug resistance, MDR, Pgp inhibitor, multi-drug resistance, breast cancer

9.1 Introduction

Raised screening and advancements in screening technologies have increased the likelihood that breast cancer will be detected at an earlier stage, allowing for more effective treatment [1, 2]. Despite significant advances in pharmacological therapy, metastatic breast cancer remains a severe malignant condition with a low cure rate [3]. Today's wide availability of treatment options might be hindered by the development of

**Corresponding author*: rishabhamalviya19@gmail.com

Rishabha Malviya, Arun Kumar Singh and Deepika Yadav. Multi-Drug Resistance in Cancer: Mechanism and Treatment Strategies, (171–194) © 2023 Scrivener Publishing LLC

drug-resistant microorganisms, known as multi-drug-resistant (MDR). In the next section, the researcher will delve into the correlation between drug efflux transporter overexpression and the MDR phenotype.

9.2 Breast Cancer Categorization and Epidemiological Studies

For females, breast cancer is the worst variety due to its high incidence and high fatality rate [1]. Every year since 2008 the number of new instances of breast cancer has increased by nearly 20%. Breast cancer accounts for around 25% of all new cancer diagnoses each year [2]. Invasive breast cancer will affect around 2,400 men and 250,000 women this year. Breast cancer may affect anybody at any time in life.

According to SEER, the median age of women diagnosed with cancer between 2010 and 2014 was 62 years old. While everybody is at risk of developing breast cancer, middle-aged women (55-64) are statistically more likely to be diagnosed. Each year, more than 70,000 people in the United States get a cancer diagnosis. Among women of childbearing age, breast cancer is the leading cause of cancer-related mortality [3, 4]. One study suggests that breast cancer kills more women than lung cancer does (the second most common disease among women). Estimates show that cancer will claim the lives of over 40,000 American women this year alone [5]. Breast cancer now claims the lives of more women than lung cancer does. Therefore, it is of the highest urgency to discover and apply novel treatments for this pervasive and fatal disease.

It is possible to classify breast cancer in several ways. It is challenging to categorize this condition due to the great variety of prognostic signs and treatment choices, as well as the pervasiveness of schemas. Histological findings are employed as a preliminary classification tool. There are many different kinds of breast cancer, in fact, over 18. Breast cancer is classified according to its stage and grade, with the three most frequent types being intraductal, *in situ* ductal, and situ lobular carcinoma. Lymph node metastasis is characteristic of stages 2 and 3, whereas metastasis to distant organs is characteristic of stage 4 [6–9]. Breast cancer has been divided into subgroups based on differences between tumor cells and tumor tissue. Tumor cells are graded on a scale from 1 to 4 based on how aberrant they seem under a microscope. Fast metastasis is characteristic of grade 4 tumors [10–12]. As the tumor expands and new abnormalities appear, for example, the risk increases. This is why it is crucial to talk about the tumor's stage and grade. Therefore, receptor status is now often considered when deciding on a treatment plan for breast cancer. Human epidermal growth factor receptor 2 (HER2), progesterone receptor (PR), and estrogen receptor (ER) are often used hormone receptors in a variety of breast cancer molecular subtypes (HER2). Breast tumors may be further subdivided into HER2-enriched tumors, basal-like tumors, and luminal A/B cell-enriched tumors [11]. The simultaneous silence of these three receptors is a hallmark of the triple-negative subtype of breast cancer. Due to its aggressiveness, propensity to metastasize, treatment challenges (more in-depth basic research is needed to identify useful oncogenic targets for effective gene therapy and combinational therapy [12]), and propensity to develop drug resistance, the triple-negative subtype of breast cancer receives a disproportionate amount of attention from researchers and clinicians despite accounting for only 10% to 20% of all cases. Recently, researchers have focused on the BRCA1 and BRCA2 genes [11]. These genes are critical contributors to the process of carcinogenesis.

9.2.1 Treatment Options for Women With Breast Cancer

The current standard of care for breast cancer treatment [13, 14] is the use of a combination of treatments (such as surgery and pharmacological therapy or surgery plus immunotherapy). After a tumor has been removed surgically from the abdomen or elsewhere, radiation therapy is commonly used to treat metastatic breast cancer in lymph nodes and other organs. Preventing, controlling, or eliminating cancer micrometastases is the goal of drug treatment, which is often used as a neoadjuvant to reduce locally progressed tumors or as an adjuvant to increase the effectiveness of surgery. Drug therapy for systemic treatment becomes more important when the main objective of advanced breast cancer treatment changes from symptom management to eradication or control of metastatic tissues.

Most experts agree that hormonal therapy, chemotherapy, and targeted medications are the best options for treating breast cancer. The histological subtype, receptor status, and expression of other molecular markers should all be considered when designing a therapeutic strategy. Tamoxifen is often used for individuals with ER+ breast cancer to inhibit the growth of the disease caused by estrogen [15]. Trastuzumab (or Herceptin), a humanized anti-HER2 monoclonal antibody, is often used to treat individuals whose tumors have tested positive for HER2. However, this progress may eventually lead to increased chemotherapy availability for more people. Chemotherapy is now the standard care for this kind of breast cancer [16, 17] due to the lack of a readily available receptor. For instance, there are several treatment options for women whose tumors are ER and HER2 positive. It includes treatments like chemotherapy, hormone replacement therapy, and other specific forms of medical intervention. Nowadays, chemotherapy is the gold standard for treating breast cancer.

9.3 Multi-Drug Resistance in Breast Cancer

9.3.1 Breast Cancer Chemoresistance

Chemotherapy with a mix of medications is often used to treat breast cancer, despite its low success rate. Treatment with tamoxifen alone increased survival from 48% to 57% [18, 19] in a trial enrolling 1477 postmenopausal women with androgens, early-stage breast cancer with impacted lymph nodes. However, it was discovered that certain patient populations did not respond well to the available treatments. The median overall survival duration for individuals with metastatic breast cancer has risen from 18 to 24 months because of the widespread availability of contemporary systemic pharmacological therapy. According to the National Cancer Institute's SEER database [20], only around 22% of patients are still alive 5 years after diagnosis, indicating that further research is needed to improve the therapeutic efficacy of chemotherapy for breast cancer. Resistance to chemotherapy for breast cancer is a major health problem [21, 22]. While "intrinsic resistance" to chemotherapy develops over time, "acquired resistance" develops if cancer cells develop the ability to reject the drug despite this. Careful medication selection that accounts for both innate and acquired drug resistance may reduce treatment failure and cancer mortality.

Hormone therapy and the newer drugs for targeted therapy, including trastuzumab, may lose their efficacy over time if the body has been weakened by chemotherapy or another treatment [23, 24]. Multiple hypotheses have been advanced to explain the evolution of drug resistance.

Cancer cell overexpression of drug efflux transporters is a well-studied and therapeutically significant phenomenon. How often does this approach get used to treat breast cancer?

9.3.2 Multi-Drug Resistance and ABC Channels in Breast Cancer

Breast cancer cells may be less effective in fighting the disease if they are able to excrete more drugs from their internal stores [25]. ABC membrane proteins play a pivotal role in mediating this process in cancer cells. Drug resistance has been linked to many different families of ABC transporters, including MDR1 (also known as ABCB1 or CD243), multi-drug resistance-related proteins (MRP) or ABCC, and breast cancer resistance proteins. One telltale sign of a tumor that is resistant to chemotherapy is an increase in the expression of these genes.

Taxanes and anthracyclines may serve as substrates for the P-gp, MRP-1, and BCRP transporters [26]. Oftentimes, these drugs are used as the first therapy for breast cancer. These drugs serve as substrates for the aforementioned ABC transporters, making their overexpression potentially problematic [27]. Substrates of these transporters include several breast cancer medications that have shown promise. Following chemotherapy, breast cancer cells that overexpress ABC transporters become resistant to the medicines [26, 28]. Especially with prolonged subtherapeutic dosing It does not matter how structurally similar the substances are; refractory tumor cells will acquire resistance to any pharmacological molecule that is a substrate of these transporters. To some extent, endoxifen, a metabolite of tamoxifen, may be metabolized by P-gp [23, 29]. Therefore, hormone treatment is ineffective for individuals with MDR breast cancer. The authors knowledge of efflux transporters in breast cancer has grown substantially during the last several years. Because of their involvement in giving chemoresistance, breast cancer stem cells have been the subject of substantial study [30]. It is now well established that overexpression of these transporters is also associated with an increased risk of developing breast cancer.

9.4 Drug Efflux Transporters in Breast Cancer

9.4.1 Exocytosis Transporters in the Stem Cell Population of Breast Cancer

Tumor stem cells have the potential to proliferate endlessly, resulting in the eventual development of all the tumor's specialized cell types [31]. Consequently, there is a greater possibility that the cancer cells would begin to multiply and spread. In other contexts, these cells may be referred to as "tumorigenic" or "tumor-initiating cells" [31].

Studies have shown that cancer stem cells disperse swiftly and ruthlessly [32].

Treatments for cancer such as chemotherapy and radiation are ineffective because they cannot eliminate the tumor's stem cells.

Stem cells in breast cancer are CD44+CD24 low/cells [31]. Making cancer stem cells resistant to chemotherapy is crucial for eradicating breast cancer. Many distinct molecular circuits have been identified. There is an upregulation of many antioxidant enzymes, such as superoxide dismutase, catalase, and glutathione peroxidase; apoptotic pathways, such as nuclear factor-kappa B; the phosphatase and tensin homolog PTEN; and DNA repair processes, such as homology-directed recombination and non-homologous end-joining. Like how maintaining high amounts of stem cell markers like p53 may help to prolong stemness. Several investigations suggest the latter is the typical situation. Stem cell-like characteristics were seen in mammary gland cells of transgenic mice that overexpressed P-gp and BCRP. For this reason, these cells exhibit enhanced resistance to chemo and hormone treatment in comparison to other breast cancer cell lines characterized by high levels of BCRP [33, 34]. The emergence of drug efflux as a contributor to chemoresistance [32] is just one of many considerations that must be made when using the targeted treatment for breast cancer; without properly regulating the repopulation of breast cancer stem cells, successful pharmacological therapy without recurrence is unlikely.

9.4.2 Drug Efflux Channel Upregulation in Breast Cancer

In breast tissue, for instance, the PI3K/Akt pathway controls both cell cycle progression and necrosis [35]. Over the course of the past several years, evidence has collected connecting PI3K/Akt pathway changes to a wide variety of cancers, including breast cancer. Seventy percent of breast cancer tumors have an aberrant pathway [36]. This occurs in tumors of all breast cancer subtypes. Inhibiting the PI3K/Akt pathway has the unintended consequence of raising P-gp expression.

Researchers have linked chemoresistance to increased levels of apoptosis-inhibiting protein survivin [37]. Due to the prevalence of this strategy among breast tumors, therapeutic drugs have been developed to combat it. Buparelisib, teselisib, alpelisib, everolimus, and MK-2206 are a few such drugs [38, 39].

Cancer cells in the breast that are resistant to chemotherapy have been connected to the Wnt/-catenin pathway, which is responsible for the efflux of drugs. Hung *et al.* [40] looked at how active the Wnt pathway is in cancer cells. The elevated levels of Wnt5A signaling in MCF7 and MES-SA/Dx5 cancer cell lines point to an important role for this pathway in cancer treatment resistance. The Tcf/Lef and cAMP response elements were shown to be active in transcription. Twenty-four paired pre- and post-chemotherapy breast cancer samples showed overexpression of Wnt5A, vascular endothelial growth factor, and/or cyclin B1 (ABCB1). They discovered that P-gp expression correlates with Wnt activation.

One component of the Wnt/-catenin pathway, Pygo2, has been demonstrated to promote P-gp expression [41]. This strategy reduced P-gp expression and breast cancer stem cell numbers, making the tumor more amenable to therapy. Antibodies like vantictumab and ipafricept, as well as small-molecule medicines like PRI-724 and MK0752, are all examples of medications that function by blocking the Wnt/catenin pathway [42]. The sonic hedgehog pathway has been linked to tumor development and spread (carcinogenesis) [43]. An increase in drug efflux dependent on ABC transporters has been linked to the emergence of chemoresistance, as shown by the work of SimsMourtada *et al.* [44]. Slow recovery from chemoresistance may be mitigated by inhibiting P-gp and BCRP expression during an active sonic hedgehog pathway. Two newly produced medicines, vismodegib and erismodegib [45], have showed promise in inhibiting the sonic hedgehog pathway and treating breast cancer.

In addition to the chemical mechanisms outlined above, transcription may potentially play a role in regulating drug efflux transporter expression. Most significantly, it has been shown that forkhead box protein O1 [46] regulates transcription of MRP-2 and P-gp. FoxO1 knockdown, the authors claim [47], decreased P-gp expression and doxorubicin resistance in MCF-7/ADR cells. Similar outcomes were seen when using insulin, a functional FoxO1 inactivator, to suppress P-gp expression in MCF-7/ADR cells. P-gp overexpression in chemoresistant breast cancer has been related to hyperacetylation of histone H3 at the lysine 9 residue [48, 49]. The MCF-7 cells, which are resistant to many drugs, have been seen to exhibit this behavior. Another study including women with breast cancer found similar outcomes.

Research [50] shows that drug efflux transporter activation in breast cancer cells in response to anticancer pharmacological therapy is a dynamic biological process. Breast cancer cells are protected against chemotherapy via a defence mechanism that is common in oncogenic pathways. It is not too surprising that other carcinogenic pathways may contribute to the overexpression of these transporters. Pharmacological inhibition of these transporters or pre-target intervention may prevent unwanted drug efflux.

9.4.3 Techniques for Breast Cancer MDR Reversal

Treatment options for multi-drug resistance are many, however, drug efflux transporters are the root of the problem. Several important strategies have been developed to combat drug resistance, including the direct pharmacological inhibition of drug efflux transporters with multi-drug resistance inhibitors (MDRi), the targeting of mechanisms that result in the creation

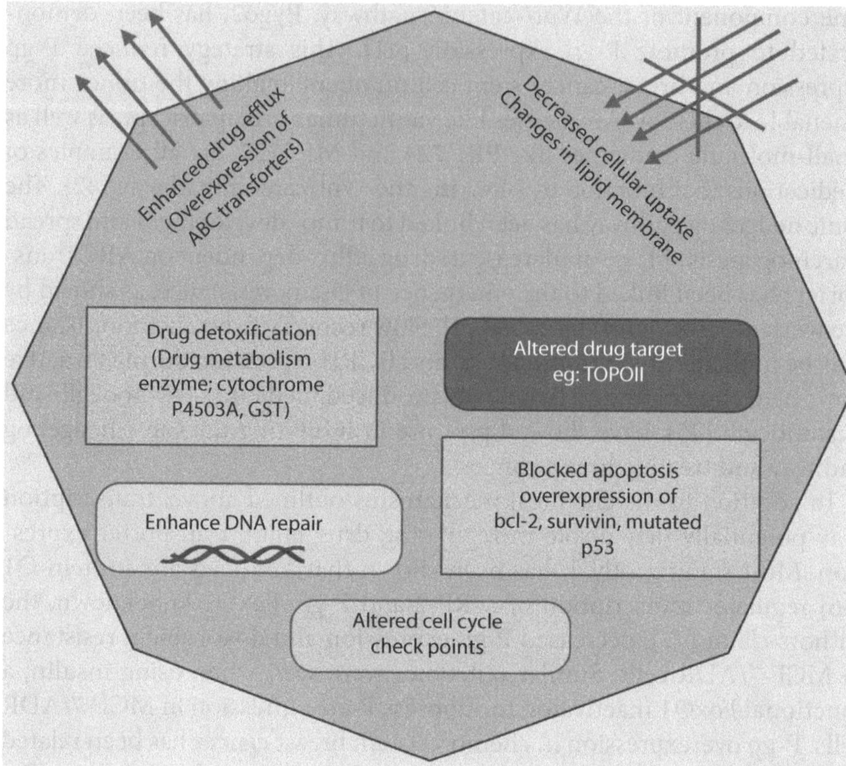

Figure 9.1 Schematic representation of the variety of methods to combat the multi-drug resistance of cancer.

or overexpression of drug efflux transporters, and the use of nanotherapeutics to bypass or inhibit these transporters. A few of these methods are shown in Figure 9.1.

9.4.4 Direct Pharmacologic Inhibition With MDR Inhibitors

Since the discovery of drug efflux transporters' pivotal involvement in the development of MDR, several approaches have been explored. MDR inhibitors and chemosensitizers are only two examples of the many titles given to the several generations of drugs used to combat multi-drug resistance [51, 52].

Studies on the initial generation of MDR inhibitors uncovered the MDR-inhibitory capabilities of some medicines that had been created for different medicinal uses. Cyclosporine A, verapamil, and quinidine have all been the subject of substantial investigation for their possible antimalarial effects [51, 53]. These medications have limited success in reversing MDR since they were not designed for chemosensitization. To achieve chemosensitization, large systemic drug concentrations are required, which is linked to greater pharmacological effectiveness but also carries the potential of unpleasant side effects. In response to these concerns, a new generation of MDR inhibitors was created, which includes drugs like Valspodar (PSC-833) and Biricodar (VX710) (VX710). Recent studies have shown that chemotherapeutic medicines may inhibit the CYP450 enzyme, although to a smaller amount than the enzyme itself [54]. It is a necessary enzyme for the metabolism of several chemotherapeutic medications. Inadvertent drug–drug interactions emerged because certain drugs were not discriminating enough to prevent blocking other ABC transporters. Third-generation MDR inhibitors were developed because second-generation MDR inhibitors had poor pharmacokinetics and few therapeutic advantages [51]. In contrast to older transporter inhibitors, modern drugs are more specific and effective. Studies in humans are ongoing and will continue to examine the efficacy of these drugs in the fight against breast cancer. The chemotherapeutic drugs doxorubicin, cyclophosphamide, and 5-fluorouracil (5-FU) are just a few that have been used in conjunction with MS-209 (CAF). Early termination of the trial [55] was caused by the lack of a statistically significant difference in the incidence of grade 3/4 adverse events between MS-209 and conventional CAF. These findings were confirmed in the third and final phase of the BMS-217380-study-01 [56]. Although enhanced drug efflux is crucial to multi-drug resistance, cancer cells may develop different chemoresistance mechanisms in response to and in order to adapt to the shifting treatment paradigms.

Many studies have shown that some third-generation MDR inhibitors might cause serious adverse effects in certain patients.

Disappointing outcomes from chemosensor clinical tests have prompted a reevaluation of the technology's potential. For this reason, a good chemosensitizer should target more than just drug efflux. More extensive testing over time is needed to determine its safety. Plant-based chemosensors have gained popularity owing to their potential benefits. Some examples include flavonoids, polyphenols, alkaloids, dietary supplements, and Traditional Chinese Medicine (TCM). Those who want to learn more might look at the reviews written by Karthikeyan *et al.* and Yu *et al.* [57, 58].

The author focused on curcumin, resveratrol, and Chinese herbal medicine since they have shown promise in combating MDR in breast cancer.

Curcumin, the active ingredient in turmeric, and similar chemicals called curcuminoids may inhibit the synthesis and activity of all three classes of ABC drug efflux transporters [59, 60]. These chemicals may affect several cellular pathways, including the well-known Janus kinase (JNK), extracellular signal-regulated kinase (ERK), and p38 kinase (p38) pathways [57, 60]. Curcumin plus mitomycin C improved cell survival in cancer cells, reduced lipid peroxidation and DNA damage, and increased sensitivity to mitomycin C [61, 62]. Due to curcumin's low solubility and instability, researchers have focused on demethoxycurcumin and bisdemethoxycurcumin instead. Demetoxycurcumin and bisdemethoxycurcumin are two additional compounds in turmeric, however, they do not have the same health advantages that curcumin does. Blocking nuclear factor-kappaB activation produced by tumor necrosis factor has been associated with curcumin, demethoxycurcumin, and bisdemethoxycurcumin [63]. Similar research has been conducted on genistein [57], a flavonoid found in many different kinds of plants. Zidovudine is an antiviral medication that decreases P-affinity gps in MCF-7 cell lines and inhibits rhodamine 123 efflux. Both azidopine and rhodamine 123 serve as substrates for P-gp. It is possible that some flavonoids found in plants might help in the fight against multi-drug resistance. The polyphenol resveratrol has been studied extensively due to its phytoestrogen characteristics. In recent years, clinical trials [64, 65] have shown that resveratrol may be useful against hormone-dependent and triple-negative breast tumors. *In vitro* studies suggest that resveratrol may inhibit the growth of drug-resistant cells. It was proven by "Kim *et al.*" [66] that resveratrol treatment reduced doxorubicin resistance in MCF7/adr and MDA-MB-231 breast cancer cells by increasing doxorubicin levels inside the cells. When resveratrol and doxorubicin were used together, a xenograft model showed a 60% reduction in tumor volume. Resveratrol's poor bioavailability and unstable *in-vivo* behavior have been major roadblocks in its quest to become a therapy for multi-drug resistance. Combination therapy with other carefully chosen chemicals, as well as the creation of soluble resveratrol mimics, have been shown to increase resveratrol's bioavailability and/or metabolism [64, 67].

Researchers have recently been interested in traditional Chinese herbal medicine due to its inexpensive cost and long history of usage. So, the researchers know that inverting an MDR is safe. The chemical components of herbal treatments, such as P-gp, MRP1, and BCRP, have been shown to have biological effects [68–73]. Artemisinin, osthole, tea polyphenols, ginsenoside Rg3, osthole, stephania tetrandra, emodin, ligustrazine, and honokiol are all examples of such chemicals. *In vitro* studies have shown that this combination of chemicals is very efficient as a transporter inhibitor. In the breast cancer cell lines MCF-7/ADR and A549/Taxol, cell cycle arrest (G2/M phase) and reduced P-gp expression were shown to enhance apoptosis [74]. Pharmacological excipients may include drugs that work to reduce the development of drug resistance. Poly (ethylene glycol)-300 (PEG-300) and Tween-80 are two compounds that have been shown to inhibit phosphoglycerate phosphorylase [75, 76]. Some researchers have hypothesized that these excipients may affect the permeability of the cell membrane and hence disrupt transporter function. However, p-glycoprotein (gp)-mediated drug efflux may fail under conditions where the cell membrane is disrupted or when there is insufficient adenosine triphosphate (ATP). Recent studies suggest that the difficulty of eliminating cancer stem cells may be diminishing. Efforts to reverse multi-drug resistance may influence ATP-binding cassette (ABC) transporters other than P-gp [77]. Understanding the function of these compounds is crucial since they are often utilized in injectable versions of weakly water-soluble medications.

9.5 Excessive Synthesis or Overexpression of Transporters for the Expulsion of Drugs

To prevent ABC transporters from forming in the first place, researchers are investigating innovative methods of controlling ABC transporter expression in addition to creating drugs that inhibit ABC transporter activity. Many studies have focused on modifying P-gp expression [78] since it is the most well-known drug efflux transporter linked to chemoresistance in breast cancer. It is possible that the use of RNA interference (RNAi) drugs, which induce mRNA degradation, may be utilized to reduce P-gp synthesis in the body. Nanocarriers are often used to carry RNAi drugs like siRNA and shRNA since they are not particularly stable *in vivo* and have difficulty crossing cell membranes [79].

The following nanotherapy section may provide further information on this topic. The adverse consequences of high drug efflux transporter expression may be mitigated in several ways. Downregulation of the Akt/protein kinase B/nuclear factor kappa B signaling pathway (NF) Inhibiting Akt with periforin may be effective in killing MDR breast cancer cells (Lin *et al.*, [80]). Based on the concentration-dependent experiment, the author conclude that perifosine administration of the MCF-7/ADM cell line reduces MDR through inhibiting the PI3K/Akt/NF-B pathway.

When NVP-BKM120 was used to treat three MDR breast cancer cell lines, substantial synergistic antiproliferative effects and powerful cytotoxic activities were discovered. In experiments using the chemoresistant cell model NVP-BKM120, cancer stem cell subpopulations were efficiently destroyed, and the rate at which cell spheres formed was delayed. In MDR-phenotype, chemoresistant breast cancer, indicate that addressing the PI3K/AKT/NF-B axis may promote cell apoptosis and destroy cancer stem cells. Zuo Jin Wan is a Chinese herbal remedy that has been linked to reversing P-gp-mediated drug resistance [81, 82] by blocking the PI3K/Akt/NF-kB pathway. Inhibiting the PI3K/Akt/NFB pathway has been found in several studies to increase the sensitivity of chemoresistant breast cancer cells to apoptosis. Excitingly, there is optimism that this strategy will help reduce P-gp expression.

It has been shown via extensive research that the MDR1 gene is regulated by the Wnt/-catenin signaling pathway. The Frizzled 1 protein is crucial to the normal functioning of the Wnt/-catenin signaling pathway. Knocking down Frizzled 1 in MCF-7/ADM breast cancer cells was shown to decrease P-gp expression, re-sensitize the cells to four different types of chemotherapy, and significantly lower cytoplasmic-catenin levels, as shown by Zhang *et al.* P-gp overexpression led to the development of a new kind of cancer [83, 84]. The author used the drug-resistant A2780/Taxol ovarian cancer cell line in an experiment using the PPAR-agonist rosiglitazone to decrease Wnt/catenin pathway activity. Both P-gp and Frizzled 1 protein expression levels decrease as concentration increases. Reducing Wnt/-catenin activity has been linked to an uptick in P-gp production in breast cancer and maybe other malignancies, therefore, this may provide an indirect solution.

One strategy to influence the MDR phenotype without modifying the gene itself is to focus on alternate routes. Norcantharidin is a chemical that inhibits the sonic hedgehog pathway, which suggests that it may be useful in reducing drug resistance [85, 86]. The chemotherapeutic drugs doxorubicin and vinorelbine were more effective against the breast cancer cell line MCF-7R after treatment with norcantharidin, which decreased expression of MDR-1 mRNA, P-gp protein, ABGG2 protein, and BCRP protein and increased accumulation of doxorubicin within the cells. Sonic hedgehog protein and Smoothened levels were unaffected by knocking down P-gp mRNA expression in MCF-7S and MCF-7R cells (i.e., SMO). Recent research employing MDA-MB-231 and BT-474 cells from breast cancer patients [86] demonstrate the importance of sonic hedgehog signaling in MDR. The most potent sonic hedgehog inhibitors have problems reaching their target, so keep that in mind. Because they either do not dissolve in water or can't pass through the intestinal barrier, drugs like vismodegib and norcantharidin are useless [87, 88]. They will thus need tuning of some form to realize their full potential.

However, the role of BCRP down-regulation in the MDR phenotype has been the subject of far less attention than that of P-gp. To and Tomlinson [86] studied MCF-7 and its drug-resistant subline MCF-7 FLV1000, which expresses BCRP exclusively, to test the hypothesis that PPAR agonists (telmisartan, pioglitazone, and rosiglitazone) may interact with the PTEN/PI3K/Akt pathway. It is shown that the PI3K-Akt pathway is disrupted in the MCF-7 FLV1000 cell line in response to all three PPAR agonists, as shown by BCRP's delocalization from the plasma membrane to the cytoplasm. Consequently, the authors of the researchers hypothesized that PTEN-deficient cancer cells would benefit from a roundabout method of reestablishing MDR. Wu *et al.* [89] investigated the role of progesterone in regulating BCRP expression in more depth. To a greater extent than in PR-negative MDA-MB-231 cells, progesterone suppressed BCRP mRNA and protein levels in PR-positive T47D cells. Treatment with progesterone decreased BCRP-mediated drug efflux and enhanced sensitivity to mitoxantrone, as shown by cytometric analysis [89]. These modifications may be reversible in T47D cells by using the progesterone-blocking medication RU-486. These results suggest that progesterone, via affecting BCRP transcription via the progesterone response element, may be an effective treatment for chemoresistant breast cancer that expresses the progesterone receptor.

9.6 Nanotherapeutic Approach for MDR Reversal

Nanocarriers have been shown to be effective in overcoming MDR in malignancies such as breast cancer [90–92] in a wide range of research conducted over the last decade utilizing a wide variety of materials. Strategies used to generate the anti-MDR effects of nanocarriers include nanodelivery of drug combinations (including chemosensitizers), passive and active targeting to promote drug diffusion, and circumventing the drug efflux transporters at cell membranes [93–95].

Cancer cells with multi-drug resistance (MDR) are resistant to a wide variety of chemotherapeutic treatments. By controlling drug uptake, drug detoxification, intracellular nucleophile levels, and repair of drug-induced DNA damage, drug transporters such P-glycoprotein (P-gp), MRP1, MRP2, and breast cancer resistance protein (BCR-P) play a role in the emergence of MDR (BCRP). Nanoassemblies have been proposed as a potential treatment for cancer cells that have developed resistance to standard therapies [96, 97]. For example, dendrimers, liposomes, and micelles are all examples of nanoparticles that are insoluble in water. Combining nanocarriers with existing cancer therapies has the potential to significantly advance the area. Multiple activities, a greater therapeutic index, and less dependence on the ABC-transporter-driven drug efflux mechanism are only a few of the advantages of targeted delivery to tumors or the cancer microenvironment. The addition of tumor-specific nanocarriers to conventional or combination chemotherapy has been found to improve patient outcomes [97–100]. When many therapies are administered at once, there is less likelihood of side effects, less risk that the therapy will not reach the tumor, and less likelihood that the tumor will acquire resistance to the drugs. This study aims to identify and characterize nano-drug delivery strategies that either circumvent or make advantage of this drug efflux pump mechanism in order to overcome multi-drug resistance. Techniques include suppressing ceramide production and gene expression of Bcl-2 and HIF1. Combining a cytotoxic medicine with a molecular targeting agent, a chemosensitizing agent, and imaging guidance has been shown to increase cancer localization and treatment while reducing undesired effects. In order to treat MDR, scientists are thinking of using a medicine in conjunction with thermal/ultrasound/photodynamic therapy.

9.7 Breast Cancer's MDR Cure Problems and Future Outlook

Numerous questions concerning the treatment of chemoresistant breast cancer remain unsolved, despite the many possible lines of attack on the MDR linked to high drug efflux transporter expression. When many MDR-reversal medications need to be administered simultaneously, controlling the possibility of adverse drug–drug interactions is only one of many challenges that must be surmounted. Because of this, many of the unwanted effects of these drugs are not uncovered until late in the clinical trial process [101–105]. Although not the only cause of multi-drug resistance, activation of drug efflux transporters is a common one. The low therapeutic effectiveness of MDR reversal therapies is due to the lack of other chemosensitizing treatments targeting other systems.

Some research suggests that including foods and drinks rich in phytoconstituents may mitigate the severity of drug-related side effects and interactions. Even though many medications have favorable safety profiles when used as advised, there is always the potential of an unfavorable drug interaction. Taking antidepressants, anticoagulants, antibiotics, chemotherapeutic drugs, or antihistamines while taking curcumin requires constant monitoring due to the possibility of pharmacokinetic abnormalities, such as alterations in Cmax and AUC. This approach is not often employed in the treatment of breast cancer because of a number of factors, including theoretical difficulties in overcoming drug resistance and the widespread use of drugs with low effectiveness. Nanocarriers may be able to address this issue by increasing drug concentrations within tumors while reducing systemic toxicity via passive and/or active targeting. There is a pressing need for research on nanocarriers that can transport cytotoxic and MDR-reversing medicines. Though promising, nanomedicine is not without its limitations. Despite the encouraging outcomes seen when using nanocarriers for co-delivery, their scalability, reproducibility, and stability have been questioned [91, 92]. The potentially beneficial field of nanomedicine has been clouded by toxicity concerns, notably concerning immunogenicity and the accidental dispersion and deposition of nanoparticles. In addition to stability, cost-effectiveness, and safety, therapeutic value is also required for the approval of complex formulations. Breast cancer tends to develop in soft tissues, therefore, anticancer medications have a harder time reaching the illness than they would if it developed in a harder-to-reach organ like bone, lung, liver, or brain [9]. Because of this, there is a pressing need for nanoformulations that can achieve all of these ends with minimal side effects. Improving nanomedicine for breast cancer requires knowledge of pharmacokinetics, toxicity, immunology, and oncology [106].

Despite the promising features of anti-MDR drugs, particularly natural items, and pharmaceutical excipients, little is known about them for use in chemoresistant malignancies. There were promising findings from preliminary research using smaller animals and *in vitro*. Because of this intrinsic variety, a novel therapy that is effective against one subtype of breast cancer may have little to no effect on other subtypes. The efficacy and safety of these medications in the treatment of breast cancer need to be determined via more preclinical and clinical studies.

9.8 Conclusion

Multi-drug resistance (MDR) is a significant barrier to treating metastatic breast cancer, however, despite the development of various medications to target MDR, the hopeful laboratory results have not always translated into clinical success. Initial results from testing have been promising. Since there are many forms of breast cancer, increasing drug efflux is likely not the best course of therapy. Since using many medications together is the most efficient method of combating metastatic breast cancer, developing novel anti-MDR therapies is an absolute need. Because the MDR phenotype has been identified as one of the key obstacles in breast cancer pharmacological treatment, more investigation into the phenomena of breast cancer stem cells displaying high levels of P-gp is crucial.

References

1. Holohan, C., Van Schaeybroeck, S., Longley, D.B., Johnston, P.G., Cancer drug resistance: An evolving paradigm. *Nat. Rev. Cancer*, 13, 714–726, 2013.
2. Szakacs, G., Paterson, J.K., Ludwig, J.A., Booth-Genthe, C., Gottesman, M.M., Targeting multi-drug resistance in cancer. *Nat. Rev. Drug Discovery*, 5, 219–234, 2006.
3. Ozpolat, B., Resistance to differentiation therapy, in: *Drug Resistance in Cancer Cells*, Z.H. Siddik and K. Mehta (Eds.), pp. 233–255, Springer US, New York, NY, 2009.
4. Fan, D., Kim, S.-J., Langley, R.L., Fidler, I.J., Metastasis and drug resistance, in: *Drug Resistance in Cancer Cells*, Z.H. Siddik and K. Mehta (Eds.), pp. 21–52, Springer US, New York, NY, 2009.
5. Swanton, C., Intratumor heterogeneity: Evolution through space and time. *Cancer Res.*, 72, 4875–4882, 2012.
6. Dexter, D.L. and Leith, J.T., Tumor heterogeneity and drug resistance. *J. Clin. Oncol.*, 4, 244–257, 1986.
7. Gillet, J.P. and Gottesman, M.M., Mechanisms of multi-drug resistance in cancer. *Methods Mol. Biol.*, 596, 47–76, 2010.
8. Gottesman, M.M., Fojo, T., Bates, S.E., Multi-drug resistance in cancer: Role of ATP-dependent transporters. *Nat. Rev. Cancer*, 2, 48–58, 2002.
9. Holland, I.B., Cole, S.P., Kuchler, K., Higgins, C.F., *ABC proteins: From bacteria to man*, Academic Press, London, 2003.
10. Gottesman, M.M. and Ling, V., The molecular basis of multi-drug resistance in cancer: The early years of P-glycoprotein research. *FEBS Lett.*, 580, 998–1009, 2006.
11. Cole, S.P., Bhardwaj, G., Gerlach, J.H., Mackie, J.E., Grant, C.E., Almquist, K., Stewart, A.J., Kurz, E.U., Duncan, A.M., Deeley, R.G., Overexpression of a transporter gene in a multi-drug-resistant human lung cancer cell line. *Science*, 258, 1650–1654, 1992.
12. Doyle, L.A., Yang, W., Abruzzo, L.V., Krogmann, T., Gao, Y., Rishi, A.K., Ross, D., A multi-drug resistance transporter from human MCF-7 breast cancer cells. *Proc. Natl. Acad. Sci. U. S. A.*, 95, 15665–15670, 1998.

13. Alvarez, M., Paull, K., Monks, A., Hose, C., Lee, J.S., Weinstein, J., Grever, M., Bates, S., Fojo, T., Generation of a drug resistance profile by quantitation of mdr-1/P-glycoprotein in the cell lines of the National Cancer Institute Anticancer Drug Screen. *J. Clin. Invest.*, 95, 2205–2214, 1995.
14. Szakacs, G., Annereau, J.P., Lababidi, S., Shankavaram, U., Arciello, A., Bussey, K.J., Reinhold, W., Guo, Y., Kruh, G.D., Reimers, M., Weinstein, J.N., Gottesman, M.M., Predicting drug sensitivity and resistance: Profiling ABC transporter genes in cancer cells. *Cancer Cell*, 6, 129–137, 2004.
15. Leonard, G.D., Fojo, T., Bates, S.E., The role of ABC transporters in clinical practice. *Oncologist*, 8, 411–424, 2003.
16. Ambudkar, S.V., Dey, S., Hrycyna, C.A., Ramachandra, M., Pastan, I., Gottesman, M.M., Biochemical, cellular, and pharmacological aspects of the multi-drug transporter. *Annu. Rev. Pharmacol. Toxicol.*, 39, 361–398, 1999.
17. Sharom, F.J., The P-glycoprotein multi-drug transporter. *Essays Biochem.*, 50, 161–178, 2011.
18. Eckford, P.D. and Sharom, F.J., ABC efflux pump-based resistance to chemotherapy drugs. *Chem. Rev.*, 109, 2989–3011, 2009.
19. Darby, R.A., Callaghan, R., McMahon, R.M., P-glycoprotein inhibition: The past, the present and the future. *Curr. Drug Metab.*, 12, 722–731, 2011.
20. Amiri-Kordestani, L., Basseville, A., Kurdziel, K., Fojo, A.T., Bates, S.E., Targeting MDR in breast and lung cancer: Discriminating its potential importance from the failure of drug resistance reversal studies. *Drug Resist. Updat.*, 15, 50–61, 2012.
21. Schinkel, A.H., Smit, J.J., van Tellingen, O., Beijnen, J.H., Wagenaar, E., van Deemter, L., Mol, C.A., van der Valk, M.A., Robanus-Maandag, E.C., te Riele, H.P. *et al.*, Disruption of the mouse mdr1a P-glycoprotein gene leads to a deficiency in the blood-brain barrier and to increased sensitivity to drugs. *Cell*, 77, 491–502, 1994.
22. Fojo, A.T., Ueda, K., Slamon, D.J., Poplack, D.G., Gottesman, M.M., Pastan, I., Expression of a multi-drug-resistance gene in human tumors and tissues. *Proc. Natl. Acad. Sci. U. S. A.*, 84, 265–269, 1987.
23. Cordon-Cardo, C., O'Brien, J.P., Casals, D., Rittman-Grauer, L., Biedler, J.L., Melamed, M.R., Bertino, J.R., Multi-drug-resistance gene (P-glycoprotein) is expressed by endothelial cells at blood-brain barrier sites. *Proc. Natl. Acad. Sci. U. S. A.*, 86, 695–698, 1989.
24. Noonan, K.E., Beck, C., Holzmayer, T.A., Chin, J.E., Wunder, J.S., Andrulis, I.L., Gazdar, A.F., Willman, C.L., Griffith, B., Von Hoff, D.D. *et al.*, Quantitative analysis of MDR1 (multi-drug resistance) gene expression in human tumors by polymerase chain reaction. *Proc. Natl. Acad. Sci. U. S. A.*, 87, 7160–7164, 1990.
25. van Tellingen, O., Buckle, T., Jonker, J.W., van der Valk, M.A., Beijnen, J.H., P-glycoprotein and Mrp1 collectively protect the bone marrow from vincristine-induced toxicity *in vivo*. *Br. J. Cancer*, 89, 1776–1782, 2003.

26. Sparreboom, A., van Asperen, J., Mayer, U., Schinkel, A.H., Smit, J.W., Meijer, K., Borst, P., Nooijen, W.J., Beijnen, J.H., van Tellingen, O., Limited oral bioavailability and active epithelial excretion of paclitaxel (Taxol) caused by P-glycoprotein in the intestine. *Proc. Natl. Acad. Sci. U. S. A.*, 94, 2031–2035, 1997.
27. Borst, P. and Schinkel, A.H., P-glycoprotein ABCB1: A major player in drug handling by mammals. *J. Clin. Invest.*, 123, 4131–4133, 2013.
28. International Transporter C, Giacomini, K.M., Huang, S.M., Tweedie, D.J., Benet, L.Z., Brouwer, K.L., Chu, X., Dahlin, A., Evers, R., Fischer, V., Hillgren, K.M., Hoffmaster, K.A., Ishikawa, T., Keppler, D., Kim, R.B., Lee, C.A., Niemi, M., Polli, J.W., Sugiyama, Y., Swaan, P.W., Ware, J.A., Wright, S.H., Yee, S.W., Zamek-Gliszczynski, M.J., Zhang, L., Membrane transporters in drug development. *Nat. Rev. Drug Discovery*, 9, 215–236, 2010.
29. Aller, S.G., Yu, J., Ward, A., Weng, Y., Chittaboina, S., Zhuo, R., Harrell, P.M., Trinh, Y.T., Zhang, Q., Urbatsch, I.L., Chang, G., Structure of P-glycoprotein reveals a molecular basis for poly-specific drug binding. *Science*, 323, 1718–1722, 2009.
30. Bai, J., Swartz, D.J., Protasevich, I.I., Brouillette, C.G., Harrell, P.M., Hildebrandt, E., Gasser, B., Mattanovich, D., Ward, A., Chang, G., Urbatsch, I.L., A gene optimization strategy that enhances production of fully functional P-glycoprotein in Pichia pastoris. *PLoS One*, 6, e22577, 2011.
31. Ward, A.B., Szewczyk, P., Grimard, V., Lee, C.W., Martinez, L., Doshi, R., Caya, A., Villaluz, M., Pardon, E., Cregger, C., Swartz, D.J., Falson, P.G., Urbatsch, I.L., Govaerts, C., Steyaert, J., Chang, G., Structures of P-glycoprotein reveal its conformational flexibility and an epitope on the nucleotide-binding domain. *Proc. Natl. Acad. Sci. U. S. A.*, 110, 13386–13391, 2013.
32. Jin, M.S., Oldham, M.L., Zhang, Q., Chen, J., Crystal structure of the multidrug transporter P-glycoprotein from Caenorhabditis elegans. *Nature*, 490, 566569, 2012.
33. Esser, L., Zhou, F., Pluchino, K.M., Shiloach, J., Ma, J., Tang, W.K., Gutierrez, C., Zhang, A., Shukla, S., Madigan, J.P., Zhou, T., Kwong, P.D., Ambudkar, S.V., Gottesman, M.M., Xia, D., Structures of the multi-drug transporter P-glycoprotein reveal asymmetric ATP binding and the mechanism of polyspecificity. *J. Biol. Chem.*, 292, 446–461, 2017.
34. Szewczyk, P., Tao, H., McGrath, A.P., Villaluz, M., Rees, S.D., Lee, S.C., Doshi, R., Urbatsch, I.L., Zhang, Q., Chang, G., Snapshots of ligand entry, malleable binding and induced helical movement in P-glycoprotein. *Acta Crystallogr. D Biol. Crystallogr.*, 71, 732–741, 2015.
35. Li, J., Jaimes, K.F., Aller, S.G., Refined structures of mouse P-glycoprotein. *Protein Sci.*, 23, 34–46, 2014.
36. Katayama, K., Noguchi, K., Sugimoto, Y., Regulations of P-glycoprotein/ABCB1/MDR1 in human cancer cells. *New J. Sci.*, 2, 1–10, 2014, Article ID 476974.

37. Ward, A., Reyes, C.L., Yu, J., Roth, C.B., Chang, G., Flexibility in the ABC transporter MsbA: Alternating access with a twist. *Proc. Natl. Acad. Sci. U. S. A.*, 104, 19005–19010, 2007.
38. Dawson, R.J., Locher, K.P., Structure of a bacterial multi-drug ABC transporter. *Nature*, 443, 180–185, 2006.
39. Verhalen, B., Dastvan, R., Thangapandian, S., Peskova, Y., Koteiche, H.A., Nakamoto, R.K., Tajkhorshid, E., McHaourab, H.S., Energy transduction and alternating access of the mammalian ABC transporter P-glycoprotein. *Nature*, 543, 738–741, 2017.
40. Moeller, A., Lee, S.C., Tao, H., Speir, J.A., Chang, G., Urbatsch, I.L., Potter, C.S., Carragher, B., Zhang, Q., Distinct conformational spectrum of homologous multi-drug ABC transporters. *Structure*, 23, 450–460, 2015.
41. Kerbel, R.S., Human tumor xenografts as predictive preclinical models for anticancer drug activity in humans: Better than commonly perceived-but they can be improved. *Cancer Biol. Ther.*, 2, S134–139, 2003.
42. Caffrey, P.B. and Frenkel, G.D., Treatment of human ovarian tumor xenografts with selenite prevents the melphalan-induced development of drug resistance. *Anticancer Res.*, 18, 3017–3020, 1998.
43. Caffrey, P.B. and Frenkel, G.D., Selenium compounds prevent the induction of drug resistance by cisplatin in human ovarian tumor xenografts *in vivo*. *Cancer Chemother. Pharmacol.*, 46, 74–78, 2000.
44. Caffrey, P.B. and Frenkel, G.D., Selenite enhances and prolongs the efficacy of cisplatin treatment of human ovarian tumor xenografts. *In Vivo*, 26, 549–552, 2012.
45. Caffrey, P.B. and Frenkel, G.D., Prevention of carboplatin-induced resistance in human ovarian tumor xenografts by selenite. *Anticancer Res.*, 33, 4249–4254, 2013.
46. Glavinas, H., Krajcsi, P., Cserepes, J., Sarkadi, B., The role of ABC transporters in drug resistance, metabolism and toxicity. *Curr. Drug Deliv.*, 1, 27–42, 2004.
47. Gottesman, M.M., Fojo, T., Bates, S.E., Multi-drug resistance in cancer: Role of ATP-dependent transporters. *Nat. Rev. Cancer*, 2, 48–58, 2002.
48. Beketic-Oreskovic, L., Duran, G.E., Chen, G., Dumontet, C., Sikic, B.I., Decreased mutation rate for cellular resistance to doxorubicin and suppression of mdr1 gene activation by the cyclosporin PSC 833. *J. Natl. Cancer Inst.*, 87, 1593–1602, 1995.
49. Ogino, J., Moore, R.E., Patterson, G.M., Smith, C.D., Dendroamides, new cyclic hexapeptides from a blue-green alga. Multi-drug-resistance reversing activity of dendroamide A. *J. Nat. Prod.*, 59, 581–586, 1996.
50. Banker, R. and Carmeli, S., Tenuecyclamides A-D, cyclic hexapeptides from the cyanobacterium Nostoc spongiaeforme var. tenue. *J. Nat. Prod.*, 61, 1248–1251, 1998.

51. Fu, X., Do, T., Schmitz, F.J., Andrusevich, V., Engel, M.H., New cyclic peptides from the ascidian Lissoclinum patella. *J. Nat. Prod.*, 61, 1547–1551, 1998.
52. Callaghan, R., Luk, F., Bebawy, M., Inhibition of the multi-drug resistance P-glycoprotein: time for a change of strategy? *Drug Metab. Dispos.*, 42, 4, 623–631, 2014.
53. Tao, H., Weng, Y., Zhuo, R., Chang, G., Urbatsch, I.L., Zhang, Q., Design and synthesis of Selenazole-containing peptides for cocrystallization with P-glycoprotein. *Chembiochem*, 12, 868–873, 2011.
54. Johnson, Z.L. and Chen, J., Structural basis of substrate recognition by the multi-drug resistance protein MRP1. *Cell*, 168, 1075–1085, e1079, 2017.
55. Sharom, F.J., Complex interplay between the P-Glycoprotein multi-drug efflux pump and the membrane: Its role in modulating protein function. *Front. Oncol.*, 4, 41, 2014.
56. Pluchino, K.M., Hall, M.D., Moen, J.K., Chufan, E.E., Fetsch, P.A., Shukla, S., Gill, D.R., Hyde, S.C., Xia, D., Ambudkar, S.V., Gottesman, M.M., Human-mouse chimeras with normal expression and function reveal that major domain swapping is tolerated by P-glycoprotein (ABCB1). *Biochemistry*, 55, 10101023, 2016.
57. Kim, I.W., Booth-Genthe, C., Ambudkar, S.V., Relationship between drugs and functional activity of various mammalian P-glycoproteins (ABCB1). *Mini. Rev. Med. Chem.*, 8, 193–200, 2008.
58. Gottesman, M.M. and Pastan, I., Biochemistry of multi-drug resistance mediated by the multi-drug transporter. *Annu. Rev. Biochem.*, 62, 385–427, 1993.
59. Dey, S., Ramachandra, M., Pastan, I., Gottesman, M.M., Ambudkar, S.V., Evidence for two nonidentical drug-interaction sites in the human P-glycoprotein. *Proc. Natl. Acad. Sci. U. S. A.*, 94, 10594–10599, 1997.
60. Al-Shawi, M.K. and Omote, H., The remarkable transport mechanism of P-glycoprotein: A multi-drug transporter. *J. Bioenerg. Biomembr.*, 37, 489–496, 2005.
61. Shaffer, B.C., Gillet, J.P., Patel, C., Baer, M.R., Bates, S.E., Gottesman, M.M., Drug resistance: Still a daunting challenge to the successful treatment of AML. *Drug Resist. Update*, 15, 62–69, 2012.
62. Dean, M., Fojo, T., Bates, S., Tumour stem cells and drug resistance. *Nat. Rev. Cancer*, 5, 275–284, 2005.
63. Hollt, V., Kouba, M., Dietel, M., Vogt, G., Stereoisomers of calcium antagonists which differ markedly in their potencies as calcium blockers are equally effective in modulating drug transport by P-glycoprotein. *Biochem. Pharmacol.*, 43, 2601–2608, 1992.
64. List, A.F., Kopecky, K.J., Willman, C.L., Head, D.R., Persons, D.L., Slovak, M.L., Dorr, R., Karanes, C., Hynes, H.E., Doroshow, J.H., Shurafa, M., Appelbaum, F.R., Benefit of cyclosporine modulation of drug resistance

in patients with poor-risk acute myeloid leukemia: A Southwest Oncology Group study. *Blood*, 98, 32123220, 2001.
65. Slate, D.L., Bruno, N.A., Casey, S.M., Zutshi, N., Garvin, L.J., Wu, H., Pfister, J.R., RS-33295-198: A novel, potent modulator of P-glycoprotein-mediated multi-drug resistance. *Anticancer Res.*, 15, 811–814, 1995.
66. Martin, C., Berridge, G., Mistry, P., Higgins, C., Charlton, P., Callaghan, R., The molecular interaction of the high affinity reversal agent XR9576 with P-glycoprotein. *Br. J. Pharmacol.*, 128, 403–411, 1999.
67. Loo, T.W., Bartlett, M.C., Detty, M.R., Clarke, D.M., The ATPase activity of the P-glycoprotein drug pump is highly activated when the N-terminal and central regions of the nucleotide-binding domains are linked closely together. *J. Biol. Chem.*, 287, 26806–26816, 2012.
68. Weidner, L.D., Fung, K.L., Kannan, P., Moen, J.K., Kumar, J.S., Mulder, J., Innis, R.B., Gottesman, M.M., Hall, M.D., Tariquidar is an inhibitor and not a substrate of human and mouse P-glycoprotein. *Drug Metab. Dispos.*, 44, 275282, 2016.
69. Kannan, P., Telu, S., Shukla, S., Ambudkar, S.V., Pike, V.W., Halldin, C., Gottesman, M.M., Innis, R.B., Hall, M.D., The "specific" P-glycoprotein inhibitor Tariquidar is also a substrate and an inhibitor for breast cancer resistance protein (BCRP/ABCG2). *ACS Chem. Neurosci.*, 2, 82–89, 2011.
70. Emmert, D., Campos, C.R., Ward, D., Lu, P., Namanja, H.A., Bohn, K., Miller, D.S., Sharom, F.J., Chmielewski, J., Hrycyna, C.A., Reversible dimers of the atypical antipsychotic quetiapine inhibit p-glycoprotein-mediated efflux *in vitro* with increased binding affinity and *in situ* at the blood-brain barrier. *ACS Chem. Neurosci.*, 5, 305–317, 2014.
71. Bohn, K., Lange, A., Chmielewski, J., Hrycyna, C.A., Dual modulation of human P-glycoprotein and ABCG2 with prodrug dimers of the atypical antipsychotic agent paliperidone in a model of the blood-brain barrier. *Mol. Pharmacol.*, 14, 11071119, 2017.
72. Loo, T.W. and Clarke, D.M., Tariquidar inhibits P-glycoprotein drug efflux but activates ATPase activity by blocking transition to an open conformation. *Biochem. Pharmacol.*, 92, 558–566, 2014.
73. Abbasi, M., Lavasanifar, A., Uludag, H., Recent attempts at RNAi-mediated P-glycoprotein downregulation for reversal of multi-drug resistance in cancer. *Med. Res. Rev.*, 33, 33–53, 2013.
74. Nobili, S., Landini, I., Mazzei, T., Mini, E., Overcoming tumor multi-drug resistance using drugs able to evade P-glycoprotein or to exploit its expression. *Med. Res. Rev.*, 32, 1220–1262, 2012.
75. Wartmann, M. and Altmann, K.H., The biology and medicinal chemistry of epothilones. *Curr. Med. Chem.: Anticancer Agents*, 2, 123–148, 2002.
76. Bollag, D.M., McQueney, P.A., Zhu, J., Hensens, O., Koupal, L., Liesch, J., Goetz, M., Lazarides, E., Woods, C.M., Epothilones, a new class of microtubule-stabilizing agents with a taxol-like mechanism of action. *Cancer Res.*, 55, 2325–2333, 1995.

77. Altmann, K.H., Wartmann, M., O'Reilly, T., Epothilones and related structures–a new class of microtubule inhibitors with potent *in vivo* antitumor activity. *Biochim. Biophys. Acta*, 1470, M79–91, 2000.
78. Rak Tkaczuk, K.H., Ixabepilone as monotherapy or in combination with capecitabine for the treatment of advanced breast cancer. *Breast Cancer (Auckl)*, 5, 1–14, 2011.
79. Lee, F.Y., Borzilleri, R., Fairchild, C.R., Kamath, A., Smykla, R., Kramer, R., Vite, G., Preclinical discovery of ixabepilone, a highly active antineoplastic agent. *Cancer Chemother. Pharmacol.*, 63, 157–166, 2008.
80. Lee, F.Y., Borzilleri, R., Fairchild, C.R., Kim, S.H., Long, B.H., Reventos-Suarez, C., Vite, G.D., Rose, W.C., Kramer, R.A., BMS-247550: A novel epothilone analog with a mode of action similar to paclitaxel but possessing superior antitumor efficacy. *Clin. Cancer Res.*, 7, 1429–1437, 2001.
81. Kingston, D.G. and Newman, D.J., Taxoids: Cancer-fighting compounds from nature. *Curr. Opin. Drug Discovery Dev.*, 10, 130–144, 2007.
82. Abidi, A., Cabazitaxel: A novel taxane for metastatic castration-resistant prostate cancer-current implications and future prospects. *J. Pharmacol. Pharmacother.*, 4, 230–237, 2013.
83. Bouchet, B.P. and Galmarini, C.M., Cabazitaxel, a new taxane with favorable properties. *Drugs Today (Barc)*, 46, 735–742, 2010.
84. Vredenburg, M.R., Ojima, I., Veith, J., Pera, P., Kee, K., Cabral, F., Sharma, A., Kanter, P., Greco, W.R., Bernacki, R.J., Effects of orally active taxanes on P-glycoprotein modulation and colon and breast carcinoma drug resistance. *J. Natl. Cancer Inst.*, 93, 1234–1245, 2001.
85. Duran, G.E., Wang, Y.C., Francisco, E.B., Rose, J.C., Martinez, F.J., Coller, J., Brassard, D., Vrignaud, P., Sikic, B.I., Mechanisms of resistance to cabazitaxel. *Mol. Cancer Ther.*, 14, 193–201, 2015.
86. Ferlini, C., Distefano, M., Pignatelli, F., Lin, S., Riva, A., Bombardelli, E., Mancuso, S., Ojima, I., Scambia, G., Antitumour activity of novel taxanes that act at the same time as cytotoxic agents and P-glycoprotein inhibitors. *Br. J. Cancer*, 83, 1762–1768, 2000.
87. Sears, J.E. and Boger, D.L., Total synthesis of vinblastine, related natural products, and key analogues and development of inspired methodology suitable for the systematic study of their structure-function properties. *Acc. Chem. Res.*, 48, 653–662, 2015.
88. Voss, M.E., Ralph, J.M., Xie, D., Manning, D.D., Chen, X., Frank, A.J., Leyhane, A.J., Liu, L., Stevens, J.M., Budde, C., Surman, M.D., Friedrich, T., Peace, D., Scott, I.L., Wolf, M., Johnson, R., Synthesis and SAR of vinca alkaloid analogues. *Bioorg. Med. Chem. Lett.*, 19, 1245–1249, 2009.
89. Etievant, C., Barret, J.-M., Kruczynski, A., Perrin, D., Hill, B.T., Vinflunine (20', 20'-difluoro-3', 4'-dihydrovinorelbine), a novel Vinca alkaloid, which participates in P-glycoprotein (Pgp)-mediated multi-drug resistance *in vivo* and *in vitro*. *Invest. New Drugs*, 16, 3–17, 1998.

90. Gerullis, H., Wawroschek, F., Kohne, C.H., Ecke, T.H., Vinflunine in the treatment of advanced urothelial cancer: Clinical evidence and experience. *Ther. Adv. Urol.*, 9, 28–35, 2017.
91. Barker, T.J., Duncan, K.K., Otrubova, K., Boger, D.L., Potent vinblastine C20' ureas displaying additionally improved activity against a vinblastine-resistant cancer cell line. *ACS Med. Chem. Lett.*, 4, 985–988, 2013.
92. Carney, D.W., Lukesh, J.C. 3rd, Brody, D.M., Brutsch, M.M., Boger, D.L., Ultrapotent vinblastines in which added molecular complexity further disrupts the target tubulin dimer-dimer interface. *Proc. Natl. Acad. Sci. U. S. A.*, 113, 96919698, 2016.
93. Lukesh, J.C. 3rd, Carney, D.W., Dong, H., Cross, R.M., Shukla, V., Duncan, K.K., Yang, S., Brody, D.M., Brutsch, M.M., Radakovic, A., Boger, D.L., Vinblastine 20' amides: Synthetic analogues that maintain or improve potency and simultaneously overcome pgp-derived efflux and resistance. *J. Med. Chem.*, 60, 7591–7604, 2017.
94. Duncan, R., Polymer therapeutics as nanomedicines: New perspectives. *Curr. Opin. Biotechnol.*, 22, 492–501, 2011.
95. Ferrari, M., Cancer nanotechnology: Opportunities and challenges. *Nat. Rev. Cancer*, 5, 161–171, 2005.
96. Peer, D., Karp, J.M., Hong, S., Farokhzad, O.C., Margalit, R., Langer, R., Nanocarriers as an emerging platform for cancer therapy. *Nat. Nanotechnol.*, 2, 751–760, 2007.
97. Huang, Y., Cole, S.P., Cai, T., Cai, Y.U., Applications of nanoparticle drug delivery systems for the reversal of multi-drug resistance in cancer. *Oncol. Lett.*, 12, 11–15, 2016.
98. Shi, J., Kantoff, P.W., Wooster, R., Farokhzad, O.C., Cancer nanomedicine: Progress, challenges and opportunities. *Nat. Rev. Cancer*, 17, 20–37, 2017.
99. Goren, D., Horowitz, A.T., Tzemach, D., Tarshish, M., Zalipsky, S., Gabizon, A., Nuclear delivery of doxorubicin via folate-targeted liposomes with bypass of multi-drug-resistance efflux pump. *Clin. Cancer Res.*, 6, 1949–1957, 2000.
100. Duncan, R., Vicent, M.J., Greco, F., Nicholson, R.I., Polymer-drug conjugates: Towards a novel approach for the treatment of endrocine-related cancer. *Endocr. Relat. Cancer*, 9, 12 Suppl;1, S189–199, 2005.
101. Wong, H.L., Rauth, A.M., Bendayan, R., Manias, J.L., Ramaswamy, M., Liu, Z., Erhan, S.Z., Wu, X.Y., A new polymer-lipid hybrid nanoparticle system increases cytotoxicity of doxorubicin against multi-drug-resistant human breast cancer cells. *Pharm. Res.*, 9, 23, 1574–1585, 2006.
102. Garcion, E., Lamprecht, A., Heurtault, B., Paillard, A., Aubert-Pouessel, A., Denizot, B., Menei, P., Benoit, J.P., A new generation of anticancer, drug-loaded, colloidal vectors reverses multi-drug resistance in glioma and reduces tumor progression in rats. *Mol. Cancer Ther.*, 5, 1710–1722, 2006.
103. Sercombe, L., Veerati, T., Moheimani, F., Wu, S.Y., Sood, A.K., Hua, S., Advances and challenges of liposome assisted drug delivery. *Front. Pharmacol.*, 6, 286, 2015.

104. Danson, S., Ferry, D., Alakhov, V., Margison, J., Kerr, D., Jowle, D., Brampton, M., Halbert, G., Ranson, M., Phase I dose escalation and pharmacokinetic study of pluronic polymer-bound doxorubicin (SP1049C) in patients with advanced cancer. *Br. J. Cancer*, 90, 2085–2091, 2004.
105. Alakhova, D.Y., Zhao, Y., Li, S., Kabanov, A.V., Effect of doxorubicin/pluronic SP1049C on tumorigenicity, aggressiveness, DNA methylation and stem cell markers in murine leukemia. *PLoS One*, 8, e72238, 2013.
106. Valle, J.W., Armstrong, A., Newman, C., Alakhov, V., Pietrzynski, G., Brewer, J., Campbell, S., Corrie, P., Rowinsky, E.K., Ranson, M., A phase 2 study of SP1049C, doxorubicin in P-glycoprotein-targeting pluronics, in patients with advanced adenocarcinoma of the esophagus and gastroesophageal junction. *Invest. New Drugs*, 29, 1029–1037, 2011.

Index

Printed in the USA/Agawam, MA
September 16, 2026

910661.056